The Daily Guide to the

YOGA SŪTRAS

Bringing Ancient Wisdom to Modern Practice

With daily meditations, mantras, movement, and music

By Susan Fendler

The Daily Guide to the Yoga Sūtras
Bringing Ancient Wisdom to Modern Practice

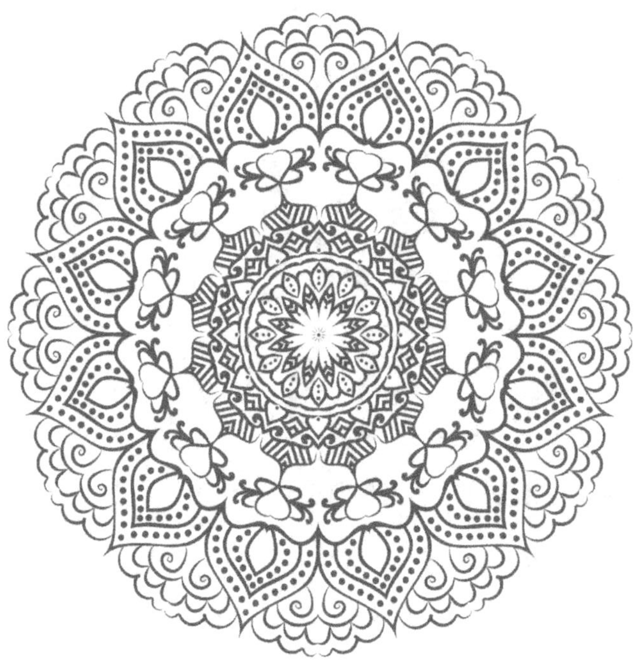

ISBN: 979-8-218-46181-2

To My Students

May *The Daily Guide to the Yoga Sūtras*
provide you with a better understanding and practice
of Patanjali's deep-grounded wisdom.

And to My Dearest Tommy

May your beautiful soul bring light to the world
wherever it manifests.

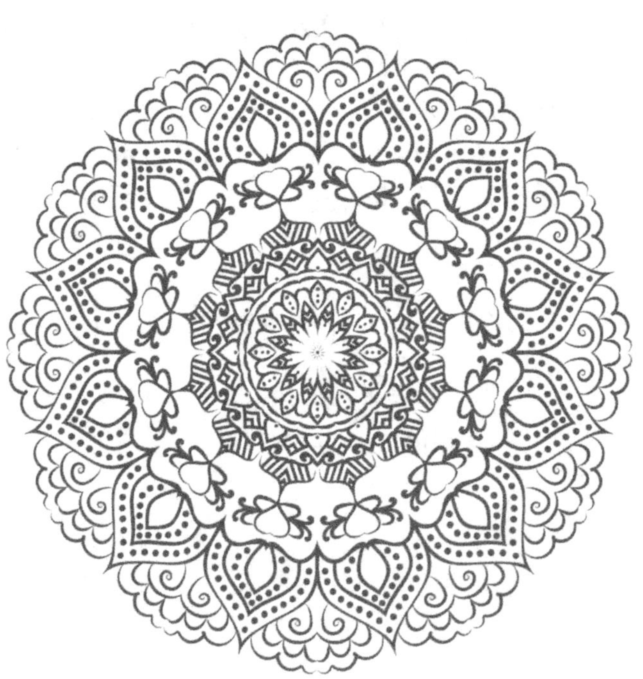

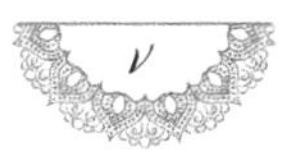

Table of Contents

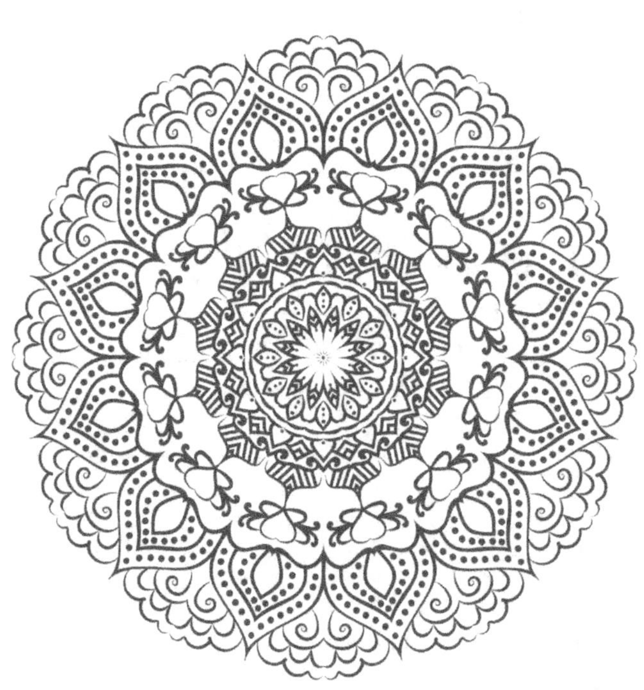

Note from the Author

I am delighted to welcome you to *The Daily Guide to the Yoga Sūtras*. As someone who has been passionate about yoga for the past 25 years, and teaching for more than a decade, I am eager to share with you the transformational power of Patanjali's deep rooted wisdom.

My journey with yoga began when my children were two- and four- years old. As a mother, I was seeking a resource for stress relief, which led me to Jon Kabat-Zinn's *Mindfulness-Based Stress Reduction* program (MBSR). Through steady, disciplined practice, I learned we all have the capacity for abundant change.

In this book my intention is to make the *yoga sūtras* accessible to everyone. While many life-changing philosophical concepts can be found in the *sūtras*, they can often feel esoteric and out of reach. I have simplified each of the *sūtras* and provided practical ways to study and absorb their wisdom.

Each page of the book follows a specific format: the Sanskrit *sūtra*, translation, explanation, and practical application. QR codes are included to connect readers to resources that will enhance practice and study. Please note that the QR codes are "active" which means they are continually updated with new meditations, mantras and movement. (My apologies if you find a QR code is not working.) In addition, the audiobook features the chanting of the sūtras with instrumentation by Alec Soderberg of All Waves and Forever. They are sung twice giving you the opportunity to learn the sūtras aurally. Traditionally this was how the sūtras were intended to be absorbed and studied. We are delighted to share this version of the book with you.

The references for the QR codes can also be found in the *Catalogue of Practices* at the back of the book. These practices are thoughtfully selected from some of the most prominent teachers of the past and present. We learn so much more working together as a collective, and I am grateful to share and celebrate the work of other yogis, philosophers, and musicians with their kind permission.

The *Daily Guide to the Yoga Sūtras* is a resource for those looking to deepen their understanding of the Sanskrit language, which is fundamental to the 5,000-year-old practice. It is important to me to share the Sanskrit language with you as it allows us to preserve and pass down the heritage of the practice. Throughout the book, I have provided each *sūtra's* most relevant Sanskrit words in bold print, noting their translations and references to the original *sūtra*. The selected words are provided in parentheses directly following the English translation, so readers can easily find the word in its original context.

As you are reading, also take note of the graphic art and how it relates to the under-lying meaning of the *sūtras*. The images will further help you to perceive, process, and retain the information presented. May the mandalas add more subtle layers of guidance.

I encourage you to use this book as a daily study guide and follow each *sūtra's* exercises. Many of the chosen practices are intentionally short, 20 minutes or less, to provide a starting point. If you enjoy them, you can follow the instructors and progress further. As you study the *sūtras*, know that putting their wisdom into daily practice is the key to self-unfolding and discovering the great abundance that has always resided within you.

With gratitude,

Susan Fendler

Introduction

The *Yoga Sūtras of Patanjali*, believed to have been written around 400 BC, is considered the most scientific text ever written on yoga.

Comprising approximately 196 short verses or threads (*sūtras*), this practical handbook presents the philosophy and practice of yoga. While there is evidence the discipline had been practiced for centuries prior, Patanjali's work is considered one of the foundational texts of modern yoga.

The *Yoga Sūtras* are not associated with a particular religion, but based on scientific principles of the time. Each *sūtra* is written in Sanskrit, literally meaning "the perfect language". By studying the sound and vibration of the words, one can begin to dive into the vibrational pulse of the body's energetic channels.

The order of the *sūtras* is meaningful and hierarchical. The threads build upon each other, and the message of each *sūtra* is shaped by and connected to the previous and subsequent *sūtras*.

The 196 *Yoga Sūtras* are organized into four books, akin to chapters, known as *pādas*.

Book I
Samādhi Pāda: Defines the ultimate goal of yoga–Enlightenment.

Book II
Sadhana Pāda: Concerns the practice of yoga.

Book III

Vibhūti Pāda: Describes the psychic powers that develop from the practice of yoga.

Book IV

Kaivalya Pāda: Concerns Absolute Oneness and Freedom.

The *Yoga Sūtras* of Patanjali is a guide to living a more purposeful and fulfilling life. It is a culmination of wisdom and practical knowledge that has been passed down for thousands of years, influencing countless generations.

Patanjali's teachings include eight limbs of yoga. (*sūtras* 2.28- 2.55) These contain ethical guidelines (*yamas*) and daily observances (*niyamas*), physical postures (*āsanas*), breath control (*prānāyāma*), sensory withdrawal (*pratyāhāra*), concentration (*dhāraṇā*), meditation (*dhyāna*), and a state of Oneness with the universe (*samādhi*).

Through regular practice of the *yamas* and *niyamas*, we learn to live in accordance with ethical principles and cultivate a sense of self-discipline and integrity. The physical postures of *āsanas* help to develop strength, flexibility, and balance in our bodies, while also promoting mental focus and concentration. *Prānāyāma* techniques teach breath regulation and how to access the calming power of the parasympathetic nervous system, leading to a greater sense of relaxation and inner peace. Empowered with these physical tools, we then learn to withdraw our senses from external distractions through *pratyāhāra*.

As we progress further on the path, we begin to concentrate our minds on a single point of focus with *dhāraṇā*, leading to deeper states of meditative practice (*dhyāna*). Ultimately, through dedicated practice, we experience *samādhi*, a state of

Oneness with the universe, where the boundaries between self and other dissolve.

In the *Yoga Sūtras*, we receive a wealth of wisdom and guidance to help us transform our beings. The beauty of the *Yoga Sūtras* lies in its accessibility. Regardless of faith or background, the *Sūtras* provide a framework for self-exploration and discovery, guiding readers toward their true nature and purpose. By embracing and practicing all eight limbs of yoga, we find freedom from suffering through equanimity. Through the practice of yoga, we unlock the limitless potential and peace that lies within us all.

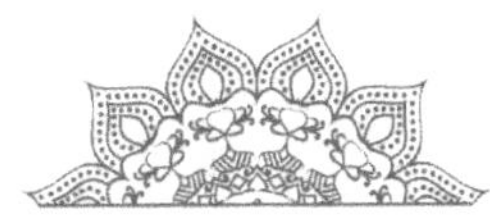

Your Sūtra Guide

Sūtra

Translation

Explanation

Reflection

Practice

2.47
*Prayatna-śaithilyānanta-**samāpatti**bhyām*

Āsana is mastered by preserving one's energy and through deep meditation (**samāpatti**).

Mastery of *āsana* comes from **samāpatti,** the harmonious union of two essential elements—conservation of energy and absorption in deep meditation. Here lies the delicate balance of effort and surrender.

Yoga refines and balances the flow of *prāna* (life force energy) in the body. However, ignorance (*avidyā*) of this essential flow leads to limitations in one's practice. If *āsana* is approached with unawareness or overexertion, the yogi may never attain the gifts of the discipline. Only when we realize that the foundation of our practice lies in the quiet stillness of a moving meditation can we soar gracefully through every pose, performing even challenging postures with ease.

Throughout practice, cherish moments of returning to the breath. Return over and over again to the gentle flow of prāna as your sanctuary and focus of meditation. Each time the mind wanders gently guide your attention back. Notice the conservation of energy as your physical body softens in response. Observe how with each conscious breath you quiet the fluctuations of the mind.

With a controlled breath, a steady and comfortable body (*sthira*), and a sweet surrender (*sukha*), practice becomes what it is meant to be—a joyful moving meditation.

Practices like Tai Chi Yoga and Vinyasa flow that focus on the breath help to find this balance. Here is a Tai Chi Yoga practice with SRMD Yoga. *(Scan QR code)*

Scan Here

You have to grow from the inside out.
None can teach you, none can make you spiritual.
There is no other teacher but your own soul.

- Swami Vivekananda -

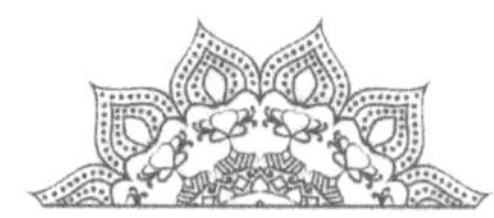

Chapter One
Samādhi Pāda
The Path to Enlightenment

Pāda One introduces us to the core principles of yoga that will guide us towards the ultimate goal of Enlightenment, or *samādhi*. It begins with a brief lesson on the psychology of the mind, followed by the commitment essential for the advancement of yoga. The Pāda concludes with a description of the stages a yogi will take on the path towards wisdom, self-discovery, and Enlightenment.

- What is Yoga? (1.2 to 1.4)

- The Vṛttis: The Five Fluctuations of the Mind (1.5 to 1.11)

- Abhyāsa and Vairāgyā: Discipline and Non-Attachment (1.12 to 1.15)

- Samādhi: The Path to Enlightenment (1.16 to 1.23)

- Īśvara: The Eternal Sound of OM (1.24 to 1.29)

- Antarāyā: Distractions Along the Path (1.30 to 1.32)

- Practices for a Peaceful Mind (1.33 to 1.40)

- Samādhi: Stages of Enlightenment (1.41 to 1.51)

1.1

atha yogānuśāsanam

Now (**atha**), the teachings of **yoga** begin.

It's as simple as that. You have found your way to *The Daily Guide to the Yoga Sūtras*. This was no accident.

Now, **atha**, let us begin.

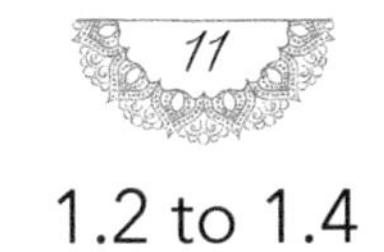

1.2 to 1.4
What is Yoga?

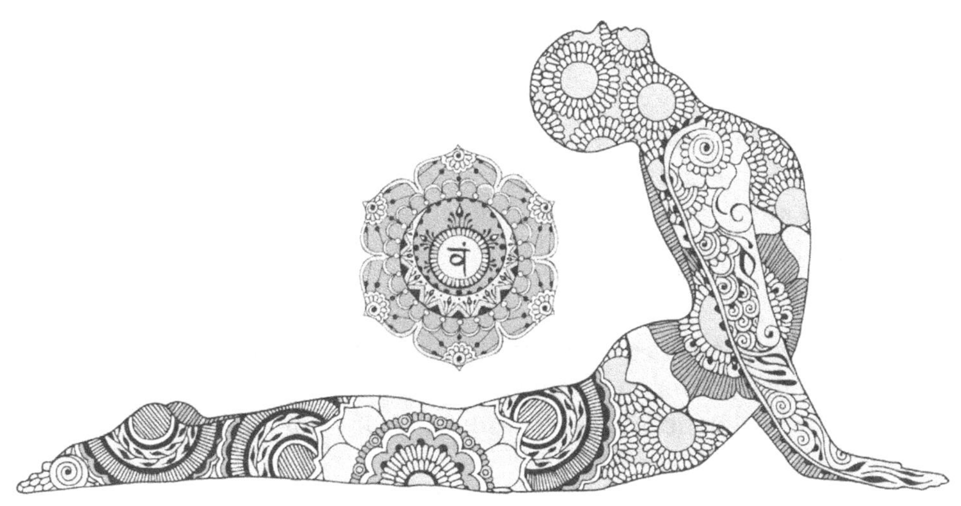

Your task is not to seek for love, but to seek and find the barriers
within yourself that you have built against it.

~ Rumi ~

1.2

yogaś citta-vṛtti-nirodhaḥ

Yoga stops (**nirodhaḥ**) the fluctuations (**vṛtti**) of the mind (**citta**).

Patanjali's *Yoga Sūtras* provide a pathway to greater joy, harmony, and equanimity. Through the practice of yoga, we free our minds from the currents of thoughts and emotions. Like a bridge crossing a turbulent river, yoga offers a passage to greater serenity and peace.

In yoga philosophy, the ceaseless inner dialogue of our mind is known as **citta-vṛtti**. Yoga guides us in taming this constant stream of thoughts and emotions, including the ones that often lead to anxiety, stress, disappointment, and grief. Patanjali's *Yoga Sūtras* provide a valuable toolbox for observing and detaching from this mental turmoil, leading us to discover a profound sense of ease, stillness, and clarity.

By learning to soften the grip of the often frenetic **citta**, we become more present in each moment. In this presence, we uncover the true richness of life. Let's begin to embrace this practical handbook and work towards a calmer state of being.

Here is a simple yet powerful one-minute practice:

Find a comfortable meditative posture and gently close your eyes. Inhale deeply as you raise your arms towards the sky, palms facing upward. As your arms descend, palms down, exhale and make a soft "ssssss" sound through your mouth, counting internally for at least six breaths. Continue for one minute, noticing how the racing currents of your mind gradually calm with each round.

1.3

*tadā draṣṭuḥ **svarūpe** 'vasthānam*

Through yoga, we discover our true nature (**svarūpe**).

Svarūpe is the purest expression of Self, our deepest essence. It represents the core of who we are, beneath all external pressures and fleeting emotions. As we explore our inner self and live in harmony with our inner truth, our **svarūpe** gradually reveals itself.

For those yearning for identity and direction, yoga serves as a practical guide to self-discovery. Each step along this sacred path is an opportunity to bask in the brilliance of our authentic nature. The practice deepens our understanding of our values, desires, and goals, and empowers us to navigate life with clarity and insight.

This journey is the heart of yoga, continually guiding us towards the radiant core of our being. Take a moment to ponder and ask yourself:

"Who am I?" What is the initial response that arises within you? If you were to ask your physical body the same question, what response would it offer? Now ask your mind and intellect: "Who am I?" Place your hands upon your heart and inquire within, "Who am I?"

Now, go deeper still and ask your soul. Imagine a warm light radiating from your heart, illuminating the depths of your inner self.

The more we practice the more we unravel the layers of our being. Through this uncovering, we discover the beautiful essence of that which was always there.

For additional insight and perspectives on the nature of Self read *I Am That* by Nisargadatta Maharaj. (*Scan QR code*)

1.4

vṛtti-sārūpyam itaratra

At other moments, we identify with the fluctuations (**vṛttis**) of the mind, and not our true Nature (**sārūpyam**).

It is our human tendency to become trapped in a limited mindset, battling harmful emotions such as anxiety, disappointment, anger, jealousy, or competitiveness. Liberating ourselves from our fear-based mentality is the first step towards becoming aware of our authentic selves, and the peace and love that resides within.

Through yoga, we learn to recognize our radiant spirit independent of our mental chatter. We gain a deeper understanding of what lies beneath the surface and flow through life's challenges with a fresh perspective that helps us tackle life's obstacles with kindness, awareness, and courage.

Take a moment to embrace the radiance of your true spirit. Find a comfortable place, close your eyes, and feel the rhythm of your breath. As you inhale, feel a gentle smile come upon you even if at first it does not feel authentic. Expand this sensation to every cell of your body as though your entire body were smiling. Revel in this sensation noticing your radiant spirit separate from your inner dialogue. Allow your emotions to flow, knowing they do not define you. Observe this tranquil space, basking in your own radiance. Shower yourself with love and kindness, accepting every part of you. Feel the warmth of self-compassion enveloping you. When you're ready, gently return to the present moment, carrying this inner glow with you.

Continue this practice with *Smile Guided Meditation* by Tara Brach. (*Scan QR code*)

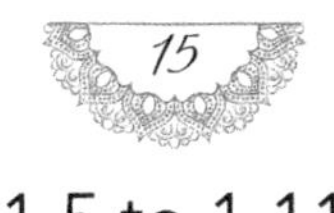

1.5 to 1.11
The Vṛttis

The Five Fluctuations of the Mind
Right Knowledge – False Knowledge – Imagination – Sleep – Memory

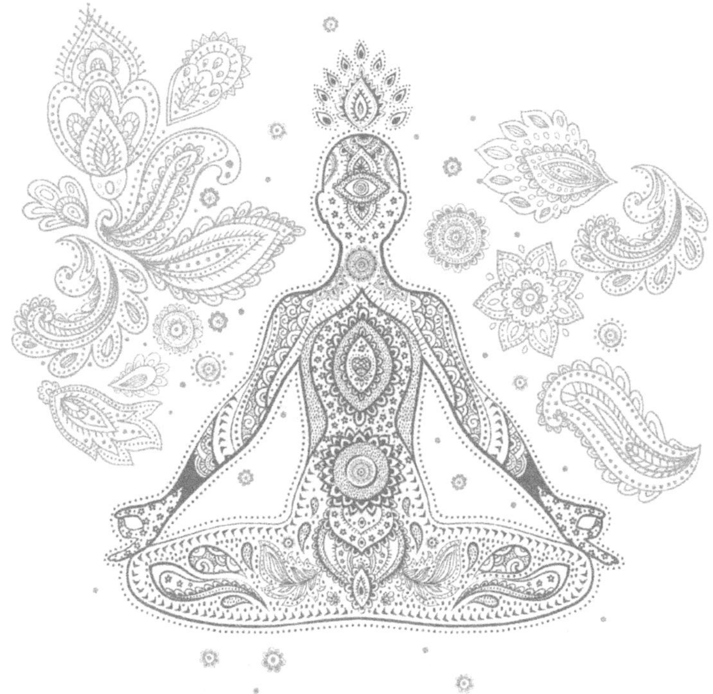

The greater part of human pain is unnecessary.
It is self-created as the unobserved mind runs your life.

– Eckhart Tolle, The Power of Now –

1.5
vṛttayaḥ pañchatayyaḥ kliṣṭākliṣṭāh

The mind experiences five (**pañcha**) types of fluctuations (**vṛittis**) which can either be painful (**kliṣṭa**) or not painful (**akliṣṭa**).

Imagine sitting by a tranquil lake, observing the water's surface. Suddenly, a stone lands, creating ripples that disturb the stillness. The ripples created by our *vṛittis* likewise obscure our view within and prevent us from fully embodying our authentic selves.

Patanjali defines five forms of mental fluctuations, the experience of which can either be difficult (**kliṣṭa**) or easy (**akliṣṭā**). Whether our thoughts and emotions feel pleasant or unpleasant, they all create ripples that impede our connection with our true selves.

Through the regular practice of yoga, we discover the empowering truth that we are not defined by our *vṛittis*, but by what lies beneath the surface. We learn to observe our minds without becoming entangled in the stories and obsessive thoughts they generate. By embracing the transformative practice of yoga, we unlock a profound sense of Self that ultimately leads to greater fulfillment in every aspect of our lives.

*Picture yourself by a serene lake, its tranquil waters reflecting the clear expanse of the sky above. Recognize the subtle ripples in your mind, the **vṛittis**, as thoughts and emotions arise. Instead of engaging with them, breathe deeply, smile and observe. Imagine these mental fluctuations as pebbles gently dropping into the lake, creating ripples that eventually dissipate. With each breath, smile and allow the ripples of your mind to calm, revealing the clarity beneath—the true essence of your being.*

Enjoy this peaceful *Lake Meditation* practice, with Jon Kabat-Zinn founder of Mindfulness-Based Stress Reduction (MBSR) to stop the fluctuations of the mind. (*Scan QR code*)

1.6
pramāṇa-viparyaya-vikalpa-nidrā-smṛtayaḥ

The five (*pañcha*) mental fluctuations include:

- **Pramāṇa:** right knowledge
- **Viparyaya:** false knowledge
- **Vikalpa**: imagination
- **Nidrā**: sleep
- **Smṛti**: memory

Mental fluctuations are a natural part of the mind. However, when we attach to our nebulous thoughts, it leads to fogginess, mental clutter, and possible delusion.

By learning to be the Witness of our thoughts rather than their director we identify and observe the *vṛittis* as they are, without judgment or attachment. Releasing the cloudiness of the mind our inner light shines freely like the radiant sun in the boundless expanse of a clear blue sky.

Find a meditative seat. As thoughts surface, label them according to the five fluctuations. Ask yourself:

- *Is this thought grounded in truth or based on misconception?*
- *Does this feeling stem from reality or imagination?*
- *Is my perception rooted in the present moment or influenced by memories or dreams from the past?*

Sit with each thought for a moment, acknowledging its presence, and then release it like a cloud passing by. Return your focus to the radiance of your inner light. Clear Your Mind from Overthinking with this practice by Great Meditation. (Scan QR code)

1.7

pratyakṣaanumānaāgamāḥ pramāṇāni

Right knowledge (**pramāṇa**) consists of sense perception (**pratyakṣa**), logic (**anumāna**), and verbal testimony (**āgama**).

Pratyakṣa, our sense perception, is the knowledge gained through what we can see, hear, touch, taste, and smell. For instance, when we come across a berry bush, we might perceive the vibrant color of the berries, and our inclination might be to taste one.

Anumāna is the knowledge gained through our logical process of analyzing, questioning, and drawing conclusions. Applying **anumāna**, we might realize that the berry bush doesn't look familiar, and through logical deduction, we decide not to eat the berries.

Agama is the knowledge gained through the wisdom and experiences of others. Whether it's the teachings found in books, the insights shared by mentors, or the wisdom passed down from generation to generation, **āgama** offers us the opportunity to tap into collective knowledge for valuable guidance. It teaches us how to navigate life and its challenges, such as how to make informed choices or recognize potential dangers in unfamiliar situations.

Through yoga, our intuition and wisdom flourish. The more we spend time in practice, the more we think clearly and logically. By immersing ourselves in **pramāṇa**, we are provided with a vast set of tools, which help guide us on our path.

Find your mindful seat and take a few moments to reflect on *what is true* with this practice called *Power to Discern* by Inner Space Meditation. (*Scan QR code*)

1.8

viparyayo *mithyā-jñānam atad-rūpa-pratishtha*

False knowledge (*viparyaya*) stems from fear.

When we ruminate over misinterpreted information, gossip, or our delusions, **vipa-ryaya** emerges. False knowledge, the second fluctuation of the mind, arises from fear, preconceived notions, and a lack of understanding.

Our world is saturated with fears and biases that distort our perception of reality. When we recognize that our thoughts and actions are shaped by **viparyaya**—false understandings based on our social conditioning—we open the door to a more expansive perspective. In identifying that we are shaped by misinformation, we find the courage to challenge our fears, face the unknown, and seize opportunities for growth.

Bring a situation to mind where your actions were molded by your pre-existing biases. Take time to reflect and journal on how fear led to beliefs that influenced your decision-making. Ask yourself:

- *When has fear or false knowledge caused me to dwell in personal suffering?*
- *How did my false belief keep me from moving forward with love in this situation?*
- *How long did I hold on to an opinion based on misinformation? When I discovered the information was untrue, how did I react?*
- *What can I do in the future to be mindful of what is not true?*

Continue reflection on this *sūtra* with the following guided meditation: *Transforming Fear* by Tara Brach. (*Scan QR code*)

1.9

*śabda-jñānānupātī vastu-śūnyo **vikalpaḥ***

***Imagination** (**vikalpa**) includes thoughts that do not correspond to an actual experience or object.*

Imagination is the third *vṛitti*. **Vikalpa** happens when we fantasize about experiences that do not align with real life. Even though daydreaming is part of a healthy creative process, it can lead to suffering when it distorts our perception.

For example, imagining scenarios of failure or rejection in social situations can create unnecessary anxiety and limit our ability to fully engage with others. Through the practice of yoga, we learn to detach ourselves from our imaginative thought patterns, and, instead, embrace whatever the universe brings our way in the Now.

When you find yourself in a state of **vikalpa,** find comfort in the following practice:

Place your hands upon your heart, and take a few deep breaths. Bring your awareness to the sensations in your body. Sense your body softening and your mind letting go. Feel your breath flowing from the soles of your feet to the crown of your head as you take a full-body inhale and a full-body exhale. Again, take a full-body inhale and a full-body exhale. Repeat this for 5 rounds. Holding onto the sense of love within, look outward, and find beauty in your surroundings, especially in the simplest of things. Savor the joy and contentment of your direct experience of the world in the present moment.

Let this *Guided Body Awareness Meditation,* by Dr. Arielle Schwartz ground you away from fantasy. (*Scan QR code*)

1.10

*abhāva-pratyayālambanā **vṛttir nidra***

Sleep (**nidra**) is a state of mind marked by an absence of conscious thought.

Sleep is the fourth **vṛtti** of the mind. Although external sensory perception is absent during sleep (**nidra**), the mind remains in an active state with internal mental processes, like dreams, memories, and subconscious thoughts. Even fast asleep, thoughts arise and pass, creating subtle waves in our consciousness.

Yoga Nidra is a guided meditation technique that induces a state of deep relaxation often referred to as "wakeful sleep." This practice reduces anxiety, facilitates a deeper level of creativity and clarity, and promotes conscious relaxation to alleviate insomnia. During Yoga Nidra practice, you are guided through a series of body scans, breath awareness, and visualizations, which help release physical and mental tension.

Find a cozy reclined position. Bring your awareness to the soles of your feet and take a full-body inhale from the soles of your feet to the crown of your head and exhale from the crown of the head back to the soles of the feet. Repeat 2 times. Next, inhale from the soles of the feet to the knees and exhale, knees back to the soles of the feet. Move to the hips and inhale soles of the feet to the hips and exhale hips back to the soles of the feet. Now inhale from the soles of the feet to the heart and exhale from the heart back to the soles of the feet. Repeat until you feel the entire body being breathed, letting go of worries as the ebb and flow of the tide of your breath washes over you.

Continue with *Bone Deep Sleep* by Jennifer Piercy, Insight Timer. (*Scan QR code*)

1.11

*anubhūta-viṣayāsampramoṣaḥ **smṛtiḥ***

Memory (**smṛti**) is the recollection of perceptions from previously lived moments.

Memory, the fifth *vṛitti,* may evoke certain emotions, trigger responses and influence our actions. With the recognition of **smṛti**, we can choose to find peace in the present moment.

As our practice evolves we become stronger *Witnesses* to our experiences and learn to sit with whatever arises, including difficult moments from the past.

Instead of allowing these emotional echoes to affect our well-being, we learn to release them through mindful practice. Through effortless awareness, we naturally let go of moments that no longer serve us, making space for healing and growth.

Sit in a meditative seat, take a few breaths and bring to mind a loved one who has passed. Think of the memories with this person and the emotions that arise: joy, sadness, grief, love, guilt, nostalgia. Whatever emotions emerge let them move through your body unleashing what comes to the surface. Whether it's tears or laughter, let all the emotions unfold. Bring your awareness to your body and notice where the feelings manifest. Guide your breath towards this area and feel its soothing massage. Now bring your awareness to your surroundings, remaining firmly rooted in the Now. This presence is your sanctuary, where you can find peace amidst the river of memories.

Engage in the practice of healing past trauma with davidji.
(*Scan QR code*)

1.12 to 1.15
Abhyāsa-Vairāgyā
Discipline and Non-attachment

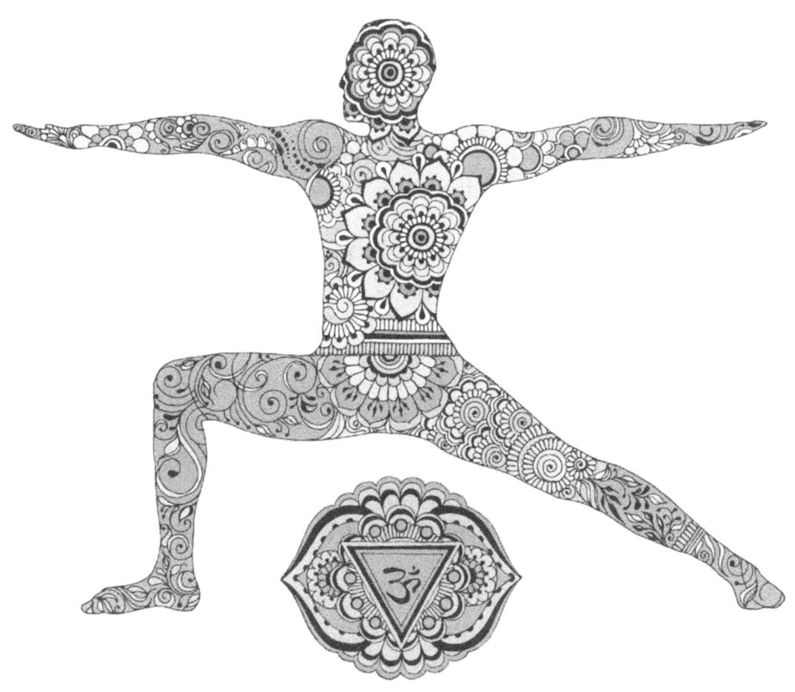

Do yoga once a week change your mind.
Do yoga twice a week change your body.
Do yoga everyday change your life.

1.12

abhyāsa-vairāgyābhyāṁ tan-nirodhaḥ

The five fluctuations of the mind are restrained with consistent, diligent practice (**abhyāsa**) and detachment (**vairāgyā**) from the material world.

Commitment and detachment form the foundation of our practice, liberating us from the mind's fluctuations. Embracing the concept of **abhyāsa-vairāgyā** involves wholeheartedly blending diligent practice (**abhyāsa**) with indifference (**vairāgyā**) towards the goals we mistakenly believe will bring us fulfillment.

Whether it's seeking mastery in challenging poses, yearning for better relation-ships, or striving for a more attractive body, **abhyāsa-vairāgyā** invites us to release our desire for certain outcomes and instead focus on the journey itself.

Genuine contentment blossoms when we dedicate ourselves to our inner as-pirations without yielding to the ego's desire for immediate or specific results. Establishing this mindset of commitment without expectation reminds us that the true treasure is found not in the coveted holy grail, but in the quest itself. True ful-fillment and lasting happiness are not found in the results, but within the steady rhythm of practice.

Dedicated commitment to yoga unfolds gradually. The first step towards consistent and genuine personal growth is to practice. Trust the transformative process and embrace your potential. Right now, take a deep breath and dedicate a few minutes to yoga.

Enjoy this practice with Shiva Rea called *Prana Vinyasa*. (*Scan QR code*)

1.13

*tatra **sthitau** yatno-ʿbhyāsaḥ*

Practice (**abhyāsa**) is the effort to establish oneself in a state of steadiness and stability (**sthitau**).

Abhyāsa takes more than showing up. Whether our practice is vigorous or gentle, it should be a time of concentrated absorption on a single point of focus, bringing our entire being into the present moment and leaving distractions behind.

To build steadiness (**sthitau**) and focus as you practice, consciously direct your gaze (**dṛṣti**) to a specific point, such as the third eye space between the eyebrows. No matter if our practice is amidst a bustling city or serene natural surroundings, a focused gaze anchors awareness and quiets the mind. So take a deep breath, and remember, if the mind starts to wander, bring the attention back to your dṛṣti.

The next time you come to your mat, try this advanced technique from the Ashtanga practice. Begin with the intention to select a specific gaze point in each pose. For example, in triangle pose, hold your gaze at the horizon, or more challenging for the neck, up at your hand. In Warrior II gaze beyond your middle finger. Observe your precision as you maintain concentrated attention. (For additional guidance to help you choose your gaze, see Appendix A for the nine dṛṣti, page 245.)

As we continue on our journey, let us take inspiration from the discipline and dedication of Pattabhi Jois, founder of Ashtanga Yoga. This *āsana* sequence is best suited for experienced practitioners, but observing the disciplined concentration holds value for all. In bearing witness to consistent effort and unwavering focus, we too cultivate the skills, strength, and grace of a steadfast yogi. *(Scan QR code)*

1.14

sa tu dīrgha-kāla-nairantarya-satkārāsevito dṛḍha-bhūmiḥ

Practice should be steadfast in its respect, sincere, and built from unshakable ground. Mastery of practice arrives over a prolonged and uninterrupted period of time.

Like a mother's steady, unwavering care for their child, we must faithfully and patiently come to our mat for self-care and nourishment. In our heartfelt commitment to improve and grow, we learn to set small realistic goals, and allow our steady practice to evolve a little bit each day.

A *saṃkalpa*, an "intention" or "resolve" is a powerful way to begin our practice with dedication, sincerity, and self-awareness. *Close your eyes and bring to mind something that you have been wanting to work towards for a long time: a personal goal, creative project, or a spiritual practice. As you visualize this goal, hold a vision in your mind of working towards it, even if only for a few minutes, at a specific time each day. Start small. As you hold this vision in your mind, repeat to yourself the following affirmation:*

"I have unshakable optimism that fuels my unwavering dedication."

Remember, real change takes time. It is with patience and steadfast dedication that we unlock our true potential.

Align your thoughts and actions with this *saṃkalpa* meditation by Omni Mindfulness. (*Scan QR code*)

1.15

*dṛṣṭānuśravika-viṣaya-vitṛṣṇasya vaśīkāra-saṁjñā **vairāgyam***

Non-attachment (**vairāgya**) is the state when one is free from cravings both seen and heard.

As human beings, we naturally become absorbed in our desires, whether they are as simple as a sweet tooth or more complicated cravings that risk our well-being. Through the process of yoga, we begin to unfold in ways that help us to observe and understand the roots of our wants. Over time, we lose our attachment to them completely.

Each time we step onto our mats we self-unfold as we quiet the **vṛttis** that cloud our minds. In learning to release, we start to make better choices. Gradually, we find freedom from our cravings and, in some cases, even dispassion of addictions. Over time, we mindfully create new, more supportive neural connections and experience deep contentment that stems from our **vairāgya**, our freedom from desire.

Reflect on these journal questions and practice **vairāgya** with this meditation by Max Baker Yoga (*Scan QR code*):

- *What attachments do I currently experience, whether it is related to food, material possessions, relationships, spiritual desires, or firm beliefs?*
- *What negative consequences do I experience from tightly grasping onto these attachments? How do they impact my well-being?*
- *What things and attachments in my life are holding me back from moving towards a place of love and joy?*
- *What do I need to let go of so that my authentic self can fully emerge?*

1.16 to 1.23
Samādhi
The Path to Enlightenment

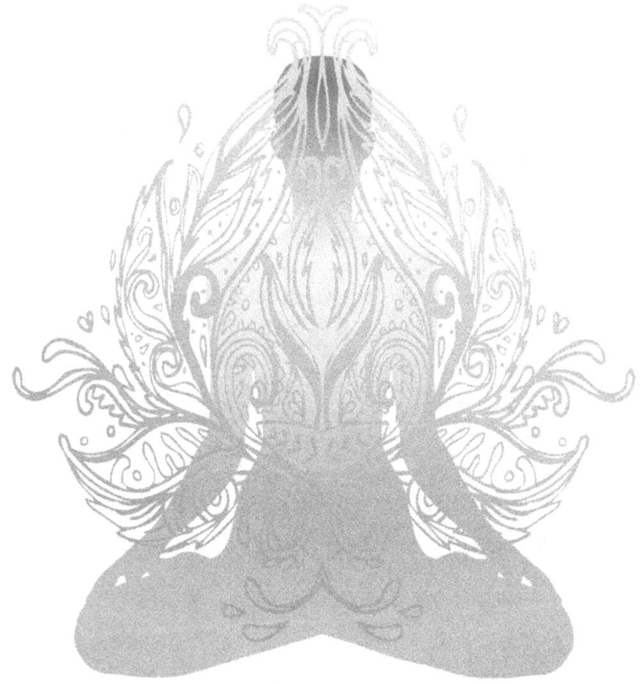

The aspirant who has attained calmness and serenity is like the infinite
sky in which storms, winds and lightning may rage but
which have no power to disturb the serenity of the infinite.

- Swami Rama -

1.16

*tat-paraṁ **puruṣa**-khyāteḥ **guṇa**-vaitṛṣṇyam*

When you know your True Spirit (**puruṣa**), then there is complete detachment from energies (**guṇas**) that are detrimental to your journey.

Guṇas are the fundamental qualities or energies that exist in everything in the universe. A primary goal of practice is to maintain a continuous equilibrium between the three **guṇas** while aspiring towards *sattva*.

Sattva is the **guṇa** of purity, clarity, and harmony. When *sattva* guides us, we experience balance, peace, compassion and joy. *Sattva* remains in a steady state with itself, while the other two forces, *rajas* and *tamas*, result in reaction.

Rajas is the energy of activity, passion, and restlessness. Under its influence, we may feel driven to pursue our goals, but it can also propel stress, anxiety, and frustration.

Tamas is the energy of inertia, inactivity and lethargy. It can make us feel unmotivated and uninspired, though it also offers the slow ease necessary for the rest and rejuvenation that ultimately instills greater *sattva*.

Understanding the complementary energies of *rajas* and *tamas* is helpful on the path to instilling *sattva* and an inner state of equilibrium. With practice, we grow less reactive, more aligned with our True Self, and more detached from the forces of the **guṇas** that hinder our journey towards *samādhi*.

Explore the gunas with this meditation by Susan Fendler and flow through a yoga practice exploring the gunas with Yoga with Shiloh. (*Scan QR code*)

1.17

*vitarka-vicārānandāsmitā-rupānugamāt **samprajñātaḥ***

Samprajñāta *samādhi arises from:*

- **Vitarka:** *Focus on a physical object*
- **Vicāra:** *Concentration on a subtle object*
- **Ananda:** *Absorption in bliss*
- **Asmitā:** *The point at which the ego and self-identity fades away opening to pure Is-Ness.*

As we begin to explore *samādhi*, we open with **samprajñātaḥ** *samādhi*, the first level of higher consciousness. **Samprajñātaḥ** is represented by four broad stages of Enlightenment, though, depending on the commentator, these can vary from 4 to 10 (or more). In this superconscious state, thoughts continue to arise, and attachment can still take hold.

Explore this meditation that moves through these first stages of *samādhi*:

*Choose a meaningful object, like a statue, plant or painting. Close your eyes, take a few deep breaths, and then open your eyes to focus on the chosen object. Start by observing its physical attributes—its shape, texture and color. Allow your awareness to merge with the object's external presence (**vitarka**). Dive deeper, noticing its subtle details and patterns, those intricacies that might have previously escaped your attention (**vicāra**).*

*Feel a sense of intimacy growing between you and the object as you explore its hidden subtleties. Imagine radiant energy from the object filling you with peace and bliss (**ananda**). Think of your object having consciousness and your connection to it (**asmitā**). When you're ready, express gratitude towards your object and gently return to the present moment, carrying peace and harmony with you, nurtured by this connection.*

(See Appendix B for the outline of stages of samādhi, page 247.)

1.18

*virāma-**pratyayābhyāsa**-pūrvaḥ **saṃskāra**-śeṣo 'nyaḥ*

The other *samādhi* (*asamprajñāta samādhi*) is preceded by a committed practice (**ābhyāsa**) of letting go of thoughts (**pratyaya**) and impressions (**saṃskāras**) so that only Enlightenment remains.

In the second category of Enlightenment, *asamprajñāta samādhi*, there is no object of concentration. It is here that the yogi finds union with the Universe. To reach this higher stage of Enlightenment, we must first go inward and master the practice of releasing our attachments to our thoughts and **saṃskāras**.

Saṃskāras are the imprints etched into our being from our past experiences. They shape our mind, intellect, and ego, and have the power to impact our physical, mental, and spiritual well-being, either positively or negatively. These impressions, whether from trauma or moments of joy, silently influence our thoughts, emotions, and actions. Recognizing the influence of **saṃskāras** is essential to self-unfoldment.

Yoga teaches breath, meditation, and concentration practices to purify and enlighten us. Over time, these practices stimulate the wisdom within to help us embrace what benefits our journey towards self-realization, and release what doesn't, so we can reach new stages of personal enlightenment. We achieve *asamprajñāta samādhi*, when we eventually release our **saṃskāras** altogether.

Committing to a daily practice, even for just five minutes, can transform our mental impressions, enabling us to refocus the mind toward peace, love, and steadiness. Today listen to this beautiful poem called *She Let Go*, which invites us to release thoughts and emotions that no longer serve us. (*Scan QR code*)

1.19

bhava-pratyayo videha-prakṛti-layānām

For some, Enlightenment is easily attained because their inherent character is of a divine nature, no longer bound to the cycle of birth and death.

Whether or not yoga comes naturally to us, the path to *samādhi* is available for all. Still, certain individuals begin their yogic journey already possessing spiritual qualities.

According to the concept of *samsāra* in Indic philosophy, beings are bound to a cycle of birth and death until they achieve *moksha*, liberation. This cycle of reincarnation is guided by our *karma*, the sum of actions and consequences from our past and present lives that set the stage for our future experiences. Through the practice of yoga, we break free from the cycle of suffering. So be kind to yourself, accepting wherever you are along the path.

As we practice yoga in this lifetime, we can draw inspiration from individuals in our lives who consistently radiate happiness and a spiritual nature. By observing their joyful essence, emulating their qualities, and channeling their calm demeanor, we too begin to outwardly reflect more kindness, compassion, and selflessness.

Think of someone in your life, whether it be a family member, friend, or spiritual teacher, who always seems to express happiness and peace. Write down qualities you notice about this person, focusing on their habits, behaviors, and attitudes. Practice emulating these qualities channeling their peaceful demeanor and character.

For further motivation read the Dalai Lama's book *The Art of Happiness*. (*Scan QR code*)

1.20

śraddhā-vīrya-smṛti-samādhi-prajñā-pūrvaka itareṣām

For others, faith (**śraddhā**), vigor (**vīrya**), memory (**smṛti**), and wisdom (**prajñā**) is the path to **samādhi**.

For some, the steps towards Enlightenment unfold through the process of building faith, stimulating vitality, nurturing a discerning memory, and cultivating self-awareness.

Our journey is fueled by our steadfast faith or **śraddhā**. It guides us, nourishes us and aligns us with the Absolute. This faith becomes the source of our **vīrya**, the inner reservoir of vigor that powers the perseverance we need to overcome obstacles and challenges. However, vitality grows not through faith alone, but also through our actions. We must have faith in ourselves to attain **vīrya**, choosing supportive practices to stimulate our health including proper diet, exercise, and rest.

The better we feel, the more clearly we see. Our new energy shapes our **smṛti**, our perception of how our memory recalls and reshapes important teachings, insights, and experiences. With this enlivened spirit, we avoid past mistakes and encounter new growth. Our faith and vitality expand too, and stimulate further involution.

Each of these principles aligns with the other to connect us with *prajñā*, our deepest wisdom. Through this process we access the insight to discern truth from falsehood, to see through illusion and delusion, and to understand the nature of reality. In *samādhi*, we meet and embody our divine Self.

Let this faith meditation, *Most Powerful Meditation on Faith,* guide you on the path to self-discovery. (*Scan QR code*)

1.21

tīvra-saṁvegānām āsannaḥ

Samādhi approaches more quickly for those who apply themselves with intensity.

1.22

mṛdu-madhyādhimātratvāt tato' pi viśeṣaḥ

But Enlightenment can be obtained through dedicated *daily* practice of mild, intermediate, or high intensity.

Patanjali emphasizes that the *frequency* of practice, rather than the intensity, is what matters for achieving Enlightenment. While the intensity of practice does speed our progress toward *samādhi*, the key lies within the regularity of our daily commitment. There is no quick fix. Rather than pushing to extremes, find a practice that consistently inspires you, engaging in it wholeheartedly with unwavering passion and dedication.

Just like brushing your teeth, commit to a daily practice. Choose a meditation, breathwork, or yoga āsana. Whatever intensity level you choose, make it a priority and commit to it daily. With dedication, samādhi is within reach.

Join Jay Shetty, author of *Think Like A Monk,* with his morning routine and 10-minute meditation. (*Scan QR code*)

1.23
Īśvara-praṇidhānād vā

Samādhi is also attainable through complete devotion (**īśvara-praṇidhānā**).

By surrendering oneself to a higher power and a deep sense of devotion, we can access a state of profound meditation and spiritual realization. This devotion is expressed in the classical Bhakti yoga, still practiced today, through asana, chanting, and dancing. Prakash—a philosophy teacher at TrigunaYoga in Rishikesh, India—shares his love of Bhakti Yoga with this beautiful message:

"The thing which I love and usually do is dance ...for me, dance is the best way to be happy, energetic, flexible, healthy calm and peaceful. If someone can dance, I believe they do not need any other exercise or meditation techniques...dance has everything in it. And it's the best medicine too. If someone is facing any kind of emotional imbalance, it's best in that situation because dance directly enters into your emotional body, detoxes and aligns it... Dance doesn't need any kind of specialization or technique. And for dance, one need not follow any religion, teacher, guide or master...so dance to expand yourself in any time in any season, in any situation... dance your way to God."

Experience the joy of devotional chanting and dance with this Mooji Mala Bhakti session in Rishikesh, India. (*Scan QR code*)

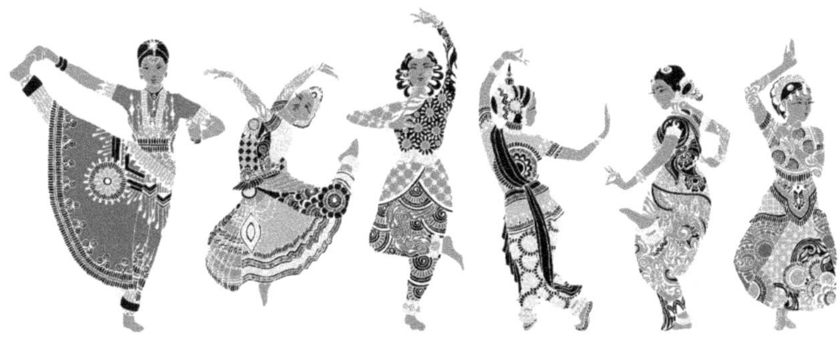

1.24 to 1.29
Īśvara
The Eternal Sound of OM

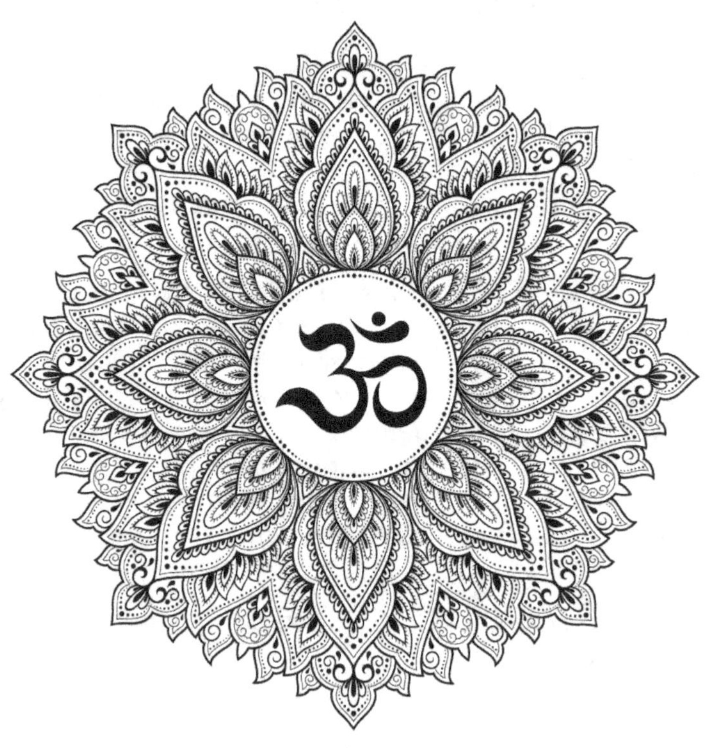

OM
The hymn of the Universe.

1.24

*kleśa-karma-vipākāśayair aparāmṛṣṭaḥ puruṣa-viśeṣa **Īśvaraḥ***

Īśvara, the Supreme Self, is a unique being who is free from afflictions (**kleśas**) and the mental impressions that inhibit the path to liberation and freedom.

1.25

*tatra niratiśāyam sarvajña-**bījam***

Īśvara's seed (**bīja**) of infinite knowledge is unsurpassable.

1.26

*pūrveṣām api **guruḥ** kālenānavacchedāt*

Īśvara is a **guru**, whose teachings are Timeless.

1.27

*tasya vācakaḥ **praṇavaḥ**.*

Īśvara is represented in the divine vibration of **OM (praṇavaḥ)** that pervades all of creation.

Īśvara, The Supreme Self, is one who is free from afflictions and mental impressions that hinder the path to liberation. Its seed of infinite knowledge is unsurpassable, and as a guru, *Īśvara's* teachings are timeless and applicable to all.

OM, the divine vibration, embodies *Īśvara's* essence and permeates all of creation. Its four parts represent the cycle of life:

- Birth (Ah)
- Life and sustenance (U)
- Death (Mmm)
- Transcendence (silence)

By embracing this cycle, we deepen our connection with the divine within ourselves and understand the eternal nature of *Īśvara's* essence.

Find a mindful seat, take a few calming breaths and begin to chant repeatedly the sound of OM. Feel the sound washing over you. Feel its vibration resonating within you, its universal resonance breathing into every cell of your being. Sense the sound connecting you to the Oneness with all that exists. Feel the limitless potential of your being, your body, a container of boundless wisdom and insight. Embrace this infinite potential, and let it be your guide, led by the timeless wisdom of Īśvara.

Allow the power of OM to unfold within you through the continuous chanting of this divine sound. Accompany your chanting with the following Spotify track. *(Scan QR code)*

1.28

*taj-**japas** tad-artha-bhāvanam*

When practicing **japa**, stay focused on the meaning of the repeating sound.

1.29

*tataḥ pratyak-cetanādhigamo' py **antarāyā**bhāvaś ca*

Through the practice of **japa,** we realize our authentic inner nature and free ourselves from obstacles (**antarāyā**).

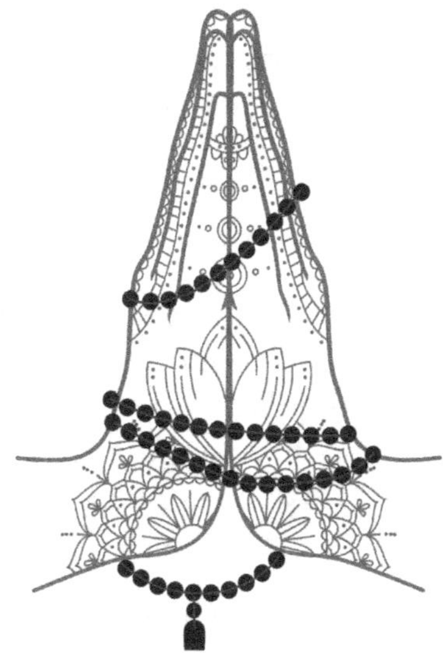

Japa is a form of meditation to connect our inner vibration with the collective OM of *Īśvara*. The practice involves the repetition of a mantra, which can range from a simple word, known as a **bīja** mantra, like *"OM"* to longer chants such as the Gayatri Mantra, which is commonly sung by Hindus at dawn. No matter the mantra, all have the vibration of OM at their core as it is the primary sound from which all sound arises.

Similar to the repetition of the Hail Mary with a rosary in Catholicism, **japa** uses mala beads to count the mantra repetitions during meditation. There are 108 beads plus the guru bead for tracking each round. Practitioners have the option to continue or reverse direction at the guru bead when starting a second round. First, the mantra is repeated aloud, next it is whispered and finally internally repeated.

By maintaining awareness of the higher meaning behind the repeated mantra, we are reminded of the sacredness and power at our foundation. Each repetition of the mantra allows for a deeper state of tranquility and peace. Immersed in soothing rhythms and frequencies, we engage less with mental distractions, transcend internal obstacles, and progress on the spiritual path.

Repeat the following mantra meaning *I bow to the Light within.*

Om Namah Shivaya, Om Namah Shivaya, Om Namah Shivaya…

Let the vibration fill your entire being, first repeating it aloud. When the mantra begins to shine in the mind, releasing all other thoughts, begin to whisper the mantra. Feel the subtleties of sound and meaning. Sense the Light illuminating within. Now internally repeat the mantra becoming one with the vibration. Let it guide you to a place of deep inner stillness and connection, where its Universal essence becomes a part of your being.

Continue the practice with this Insight Timer *Japa Meditation* by Braydon Mackenzie. (*Scan QR code*)

1.30 to 1.32

Antarāyā

Distractions Along the Path

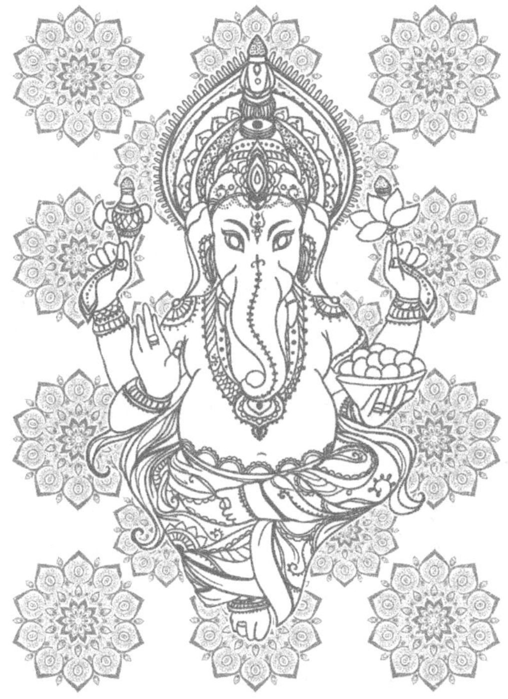

I will love the light for it shows me the way, yet I will endure
the darkness because it shows me the stars.

- Og Mandino -

1.30

*vyādhi-styāna-saṁśaya-pramādālasyāvirati-bhrānti-darśanālab-
dha-bhūmikatvānavasthitatvāni citta-vikṣepāste'ntarāyāḥ*

The hindrances (**antarāyā**) to *samādhi* include disease, idleness, doubt, carelessness, sloth, attachment, fear, inability to focus, and lack of concentration.

1.31

duḥkha-*daurmanasyāṅgam-ejayatva-śvāsa-praśvāsā vikṣepa-saha-bhuvaḥ*

Distractions may be accompanied by suffering (**duḥkha**), dejection, shaking, and irregular breathing.

1.32

*tat-pratiṣedhārtham **eka**-tattvābhyāsaḥ*

To eliminate these disturbances, practice one (**eka**) pointed focus.

Antarāyā, or hindrances, will undoubtedly present themselves as we follow the path of yoga, including:

- Disease
- Dullness
- Doubt
- Procrastination
- Laziness
- Craving
- Incorrect ideas or understanding
- Inability to achieve finer stages
- Instability

During the process, we may also experience:

- Pain
- Depression
- Shaking of the body
- Unrhythmic breathing

No matter our challenges, with practice every hindrance becomes a teacher. When we find ourselves experiencing any of these disturbances, when we feel overwhelmed and constantly like a victim, we remain in a perpetual state of fight or flight. We believe that our survival in these situations relies on controlling our external circumstances. By following the yogic path and exploring subtler states of consciousness, we gradually embrace and dissolve these disturbances. Through steadfast commitment and focus on our practice (*abhyasa*), we can release our emotional attachments and free ourselves from the cycle of suffering.

Witness the incredible benefits that unfold by immersing yourself in Jon Kabat-Zinn's 8-week free Mindfulness-Based Stress Reduction Program (MBSR). (*Scan QR code*)

1.33 to 1.40
Practices for a Peaceful Mind

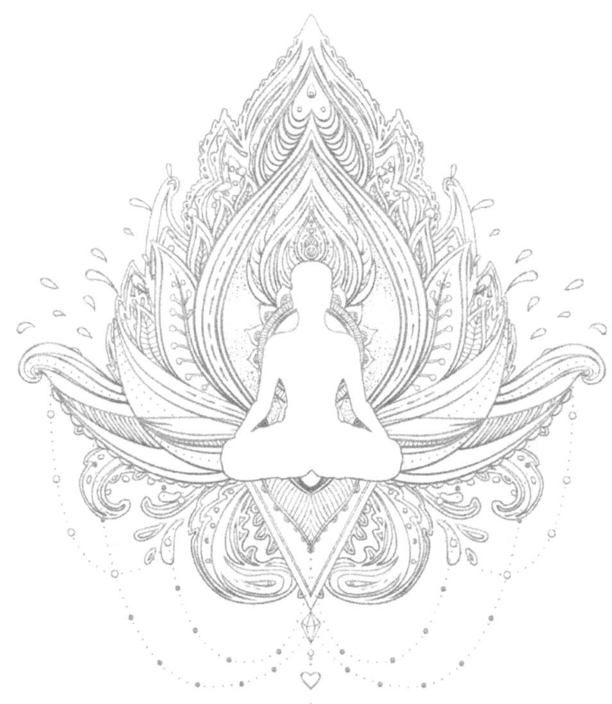

Meditation is when you empty yourself
and let the Universe come in.

- Rumi -

1.33

maitrī-karuṇā-muditopekṣāṇām sukha-duḥkha-puṇyāpuṇya-viṣayāṇām
bhāvanātaś citta-prasādanam

Be friendly (**maitrī**) to those who are happy (**sukha**), compassionate (**karuṇā**) to those who are suffering (**duḥkha**), delightful (**mudita**) to those who are virtuous, and show equanimity (**upekṣa**) to those who are wicked. This way, the mind (**citta**) will remain calm and undisturbed.

One of the first steps towards peace of mind is bringing focus to our relationships. Sri Swami Satchidananda refers to this as the *Four Keys to Happiness* - maitrī, karuṇā, mudita and upekṣa.

Find a meditative seat and bring your attention to your heart center. Imagine someone you care about deeply. Think about the qualities you appreciate in them. With maitrī (friendliness) silently repeat: "May you be happy. May you be healthy. May you live with ease." Feel the love and kindness emanating from your heart towards this person. Now, shift your focus to karuṇā, (compassion). Picture someone you know who is going through a difficult time. Visualize their struggles and challenges. Silently repeat: "May you be free from suffering. May you find peace. May you have the strength to overcome your difficulties." Feel the compassion flowing from your heart offering empathy and comfort. Next, bring your attention to mudiṭā, (joyous appreciation). Think of someone who has recently achieved something wonderful or is experiencing happiness. Visualize their success and joy. Silently repeat: "May your happiness continue, your success grow, and may you inspire others." Feel the genuine happiness for their well-being, celebrating their achievements as if they were your own. Lastly, focus on upekṣā, (equanimity). Picture someone negative or hostile towards you. Visualize them with a calm and composed mind. Repeat: "May you find peace and balance". Feel the sense of detachment, maintaining your inner calm despite their negativity.

*Continue the practice of **maitrī** with this Loving Kindness Meditation by Unearth Compassion. (Scan QR code)*

1.34

prachardana-vidhāraṇābhyāṁ vā prāṇasya

Find peace of mind through controlled exhalation (**prachardana**) and retaining the breath (**vidhāraṇābhyāṁ**)*.

When we feel overwhelmed by life's stressors, we can find solace in drawing attention to our breath. While *prānāyāma* will be discussed more fully in the next Pāda, breath is introduced here as a way to begin finding peace of mind and connection.

This introductory *prānāyāma* practice is broken down into two parts. The first step involves conscious control of the exhalation (**prachardana**). By deliberately lengthening our exhale, we release impurities along with the burdens of the mind. In the second part of the practice, the breath is held at the bottom of the exhale (**vidhāraṇābhyāṁ**) without strain or tension. In emptiness, we attune ourselves to the subtle flow of *prana* within.

Box breathing is a practice of controlled inhalation, exhalation, and retention. *Find a comfortable, mindful seat, then take a deep inhale through your nose for a count of five. Hold your breath for five counts, then exhale for five counts, and hold for five counts before starting the cycle again. Breathe in 1 - 2 - 3 - 4 - 5 - hold - 2 - 3 - 4 - 5 - exhale - 2 - 3 - 4 - 5 - hold - 2 - 3 - 4 - 5. Repeat this pattern for the duration of the practice.*

Here is a guided box breathing practice. (*Scan QR code*)

*These Sanskrit words are more commonly referred to as *recaka [pronounced rechaka]* and *kumbhaka* respectively.

1.35

viṣayavatī vā pravṛttirutpannā manasaḥ sthiti-nibandhanī

Bind steadiness (**sthiti-nibandhanī**) to the mind by concentrating on an object (**viṣaya**). Pay attention to your sensory experience as you hold focus.

Another approach to finding peace of mind is to bind (**bandha**) focus to an object. By simultaneously observing the distinct qualities of an object and bringing attention to our senses, we can cultivate a *sattvic* mind.

As we deepen our meditation practice, we awaken the dormant depths of our sensory perceptions. Classical commentators of the *Yoga Sūtras* believed that through focused practice, such as gently fixing the gaze at the tip of the nose without crossing the eyes, our sense of smell can ascend to extraordinary levels.

For a moment, shift your awareness away from this text and tune into your senses. Feel the support of the earth beneath your sit bones, and fully connect with the grounding sensation. Notice the sounds around you, near and far, and immerse yourself in the symphony of the present moment. Take a mindful pause to taste the flavors in your mouth, and savor each sensation. As you softly gaze at your surroundings, observe something beautiful in your presence.

Now, gently close your eyes and envision a vast movie screen before you. Observe with curiosity what arises within your mind's eye. Do vivid colors unfold before you? Do images emerge? As you witness these mental creations, remember you are the conscious Observer, distinct from the fluctuations of your thoughts.

Enjoy this *Sensory Awareness Meditation* by Meditations and Soundscapes. (*Scan QR code*)

1.36

viśokā vā jyotiṣmatī

Steady the mind on the brilliant luminosity (**jyoti**) within, which exists beyond all pain and suffering.

Joyti is our inner radiance and when we meditate on this light within it brings deep serenity. This luminosity is our inner sanctuary, a place beyond the turbulence of life's challenges. Within this space, our worries and troubles dissolve, and the mind finds peace from suffering as its chatter subsides.

In this pursuit, we can draw inspiration from the transformative journey of MC Yogi, whose own story of overcoming challenges through yoga is beautifully recounted in his book *Spiritual Graffiti*. MC Yogi's life reflects the power of connecting with one's inner light to navigate the darkest of times and emerge with wisdom, strength, and grace.

Gently close your eyes and envision a luminous light emanating from the center of your heart, like the radiant sun (sūrya). Imagine this golden light extending its rays like a lighthouse to the periphery of your body and beyond. With each breath, allow this inner brilliance to grow brighter, expanding and permeating every fiber of your being. Feel the warmth and comfort of this light as it envelopes you soothing every muscle and quieting every thought. Visualize this light expanding to the vastness of the cosmos. Let this warmth be a beacon that transports you to a state of tranquility and serenity, where all worries and troubles dissolve.

Continue to immerse yourself in your radiant light with this **jyoti** meditation and enjoy the brilliance of MC Yogi's *Light House and Light of Your Grace (Beloved Mooji Baba)*. *(Scan QR code)*

1.37

*vīta-**rāga**-viṣayam vā cittam*

Concentrate on a saint, a guru, or a person who is free from the bondage of desire (**rāga**).

Think of a spiritual figure who has relinquished their attachment to personal desires, perhaps Gandhi, Mother Teresa, Swami Rama or Thich Nhat Hanh. Visualize their peaceful nature, contemplate their teachings, and focus on the qualities you most admire in them. Study their work and the practices they followed to achieve spiritual liberation. By modeling after their example, we can deepen our own spiritual practice and develop greater inner peace and serenity.

Close your eyes and take a few deep, cleansing breaths. As you settle into stillness, bring to mind your admired spiritual figure. Visualize this person in your mind's eye, surrounded by an aura of tranquility and wisdom. Picture this person engaged in acts of compassion or teachings that have touched the hearts of many. Imagine this person's presence filling the space around you with an indescribable sense of serenity.

Now, contemplate the qualities and virtues that draw you to this figure—their unwavering dedication to truth, their boundless love for humanity, and their selflessness and humility. Feeling their aura close within your heart, allow their essence and wisdom to merge with your own being. Feel how these qualities begin to resonate within you and awaken inner peace. Embody your guru's aura as you go about your day.

Read *Peace is Every Step* by Thich Nhat Hanh. (*Scan QR code*)

1.38

*svapna-**nidrā**-jñānālambanaṁ vā*

Consider the wisdom revealed by your dreams and restorative sleep (**nidra**).

As we consistently engage in concentration and meditative practices, we may find that we begin to recall our dreams more frequently. Take time to focus on the uplifting dreams you remember from sleep and notice any emotions that arise. Concentrate on their deeper meanings, as this can provide valuable insights into our subconscious mind.

In addition to exploring our dreams, we can also practice conscious relaxation. As mentioned in sūtra 1.10, the practice of Yoga Nidra involves lying down and following a series of instructions that lead to a deeply relaxed state while remaining aware of our surroundings. By incorporating Yoga Nidra into our routine, we deepen our understanding of the mind-body connection promoting inner peace and deep sleep.

Additionally, we can focus on the act of sleep itself. Notice how effortlessly you enter into a relaxed and mindful state when you fully surrender and focus on the process of falling asleep. Imagine yourself gently floating into a peaceful slumber, let each breath become slower and deeper. Feel the body becoming heavy and relaxed and your mind quiet as you drift into a serene and restorative sleep.

Enter a state of bliss and rejuvenation as you listen to *Calming Yoga Nidra* guided by Tamara Skyhawk (Verma). (*Scan QR code*)

1.39
*Yathābhimata-**dhyānā**d vā*

Meditate (**dhyāna**) on whatever pleases you.

Dhyāna is the practice of meditation that will further be explored in Pāda Three. Meditation guides us to release our attention from the distractions around us, and instead focus on something that truly inspires pleasure.

Meditation does not have to take the form of a solemn seat. As we awaken to the beauty of the present, any activity can be a meditation. Whether it is eating, doing the dishes, talking to a friend, dancing or playing an instrument, when we bring awareness into everything we do, and we bring meditation into each and every moment, yoga becomes a lifestyle.

Select an object or activity that brings you joy as your focus of meditation. It could be a physical object, such as a statue or a flower, or something more abstract like a feeling, an intention, or your breath. If you love to dance, you may turn on your favorite music and close your eyes, embodying the flow of moments. Once you have chosen your object or activity, find a quiet place and spend five to 20 minutes in total focus on it. As you become more absorbed, notice how thoughts and distractions disappear. When your mind wanders, gently bring your attention back and refocus on what inspires you.

Remember, the goal of meditation is not to achieve any particular outcome or result, but simply to be fully immersed in the present moment.

Enjoy this guided flower meditation with Thich Nhat Hanh.
(*Scan QR code*)

1.40

paramāṇu-parama-mahattvānto 'sya vaśīkāraḥ

When meditation matures, the yogi's mastery of focus reaches from the smallest atom to the entirety of the universe.

The journey towards mastery of meditation is part of a gradual progression on the path to *samādhi*. Patanjali offers techniques in the previous *sūtras* for attaining inner peace and steadying the mind. These practices empower us to direct our attention towards anything, whether it be as minuscule as an atom or as expansive as the universe.

With this immense inner focus and concentration, we gain the ability to navigate any challenge, irrespective of its magnitude. We learn to become less reactive, and even in the face of life's most complex and immense challenges, the yogi's presence makes life's situations easier instead of more complicated. This is only possible through the cultivation of wisdom in our practice of deep inner focus and reflection.

Find a meditative seat and take a few calming breaths. Feel the soothing rhythms of your inhalation and exhalation, notice any vṛttis, and bring your attention to the Now—Atha. Imagine the tiniest cell within your body. Hold your focus here no matter what arises. Let that go, and now imagine the infinite expanse of the universe. Embody a sense of "ahhh" picturing swirling galaxies, stars and cosmic wonder. Hold your attention here. Imagine the entire universe inside you and let this sense of Oneness fill you completely.

Join davidji as he guides you on a journey with *I Am the Universe*. (*Scan QR code*)

1.41 to 1.51
Samādhi
Stages of Enlightenment

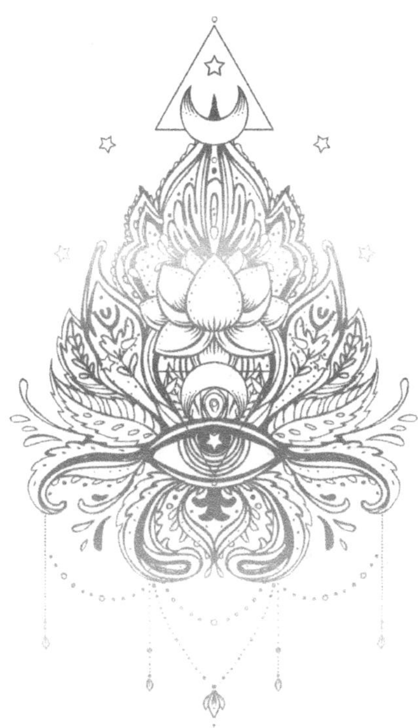

When you can quiet the fluctuations of your mind and drift into stillness
and silence, you can finally hear the whispers of your heart.

- davidji -

1.41

kṣīṇa-vṛtter abhijātasyeva maṇer grahītṛ-grahaṇa-grāhyeṣu
tatsthatad-añjanatā **samāpattiḥ**

When the fluctuations of the mind subside, the mind becomes completely absorbed (**samāpatti**). Like an object reflected in a pure crystal, a deep immersion is formed between the meditator, the practice of meditation, and the object of meditation.

Imagine a serene mountain lake, its crystal-clear surface mirroring the majestic surroundings. See the perfect reflection of the sky, mountains, and trees illuminated on the lake's surface.

Visualize yourself merging with the tranquil lake. Feel the connection forming between you and the pristine clarity of its waters. Like the lake effortlessly mirrors its surroundings, sense yourself effortlessly reflecting the beauty and serenity of this scene. Feel the boundaries dissolve as unity arises merging you, as the meditator, the act of meditation and your object of focus into a harmonious whole. Let go of any sense of separation. Just as the lake and its reflections blend into one seamless whole, sense this unity within yourself. This is samāpatti – a state of complete absorption where boundaries dissolve, and you sense the deep connection with everything around you.

Allow yourself to rest in this state of harmony and unity for a few moments, soaking in the peace and stillness. As you gradually bring your meditation to a close, carry this sense of Oneness and tranquility with you into your day.

Go deeper into your practice with *Illusion Itself is Illusory* by Samaneri Jayasāra. (*Scan QR code*)

1.42

tatra śabdārtha-jñāna-vikalpaiḥ saṁkīrṇā savitarkā-samāpattiḥ

Savitarkā *samādhi* is absorption with physical awareness; meditation is practiced on an object with an underlying conception (**vikalpa**) of the name (**śabda**), meaning (**ārtha**), and understanding of the object itself (**jñāna**).

During the initial stages of *samādhi,* the mind will still experience fluctuations. For instance, focusing on a candle flame as the object of meditation, we retain awareness of its name, "candle" or "flame," contemplate its qualities such as brightness, movement, and warmth, and have an understanding of what a candle flame represents.

Trataka, or candle gazing meditation, is a technique that builds focus and heightened awareness. Through regular practice, the mind becomes absorbed in the object, leading to deeper concentration and higher stages of *samādhi:*

Begin by lighting a candle as the focal point and gently fix your gaze on the flame. Observe its shape, brightness, movement and color. Try not to blink and instead allow your eyes to soften and relax. Let your attention be fully absorbed by the gentle fiery dance. As you continue to gaze at the candle flame, notice any thoughts or distractions that arise in your mind. Acknowledge them without judgment and continue to gently bring your focus back to the flame.

Continue your practice of **savitarkā samādhi** with this Meditation: *Candle Gazing Practice* by Susi Amendola, Insight Timer. (*Scan QR code*)

1.43

smṛti-pariśuddhau svarūpa-śūnyevārtha-mātra-nirbhāsā nirvitarkā

In **nirvitarkā** *samādhi*, the memory (**smṛti**) becomes clear and pure, the mind is empty (**śunya**), and the object of focus shines in its true nature (**svarūpe**). The object now shines in its own right.

During the second stage of *samprajñāta samādhi,* the practice of meditative absorption remains the same, but there is no longer awareness of *śabdārtha-jñāna*—the name, meaning, and understanding of the object. Now the object exists simply in its own right, its subtleties revealed.

Nirvitarkā *samādhi* is only attainable with a concentrated and glorious meditative study of the intricacies of the object itself. With unwavering practice, we gradually extend our capacity to remain in this luminous state of meditative absorption before external or internal distractions draw our focus back.

Close your eyes, place your hands upon your heart and take a few deep calming breaths. Begin to explore the sacred space of your heart—its warmth, the reassuring, gentle rhythm of your heartbeat, and the sense of compassion it holds. Feel the wonder and curiosity of your heart. Embrace your heart like a close friend, sensing its wisdom.

As your mind becomes still and thoughts fade away, allow the heart to reveal its essence beyond words and concepts. Feel yourself becoming One with your heart space, savoring the subtleties of its existence.

Enhance your focus and concentration with this *Anahata Dharana Meditation.* (Scan QR code)

1.44

*etayaiva **savicārā nirvicārā** cha **sūkṣma-viṣaya** vyākhyātā*

Savicārā (with reflection) and **nirvicārā** (without reflection) on the subtle qualities of the object (**sūkṣma-viṣaya**) are the third and fourth stages of *samādhi*. The practices are similar to those of *nirvitarkā*.

Through each stage, the practice of *samādhi* does not significantly change on the outside. It is our inward experience and our ability to perceive that shifts dramatically.

In **savicārā** *samādhi,* the third stage of meditative absorption, the focus of the practice is directed to the subtle aspects of the object like its spatial, causal, and temporal attributes, rather than its gross physical qualities. The meditator still remains aware of the thoughts and contemplation around the subtle energies of the object of focus.

The fourth stage, **nirvicārā** takes place without awareness or mental activity. *Samādhi* is focused on the object without any past impressions, allowing the meditator to transcend the limitations of time and space to become completely absorbed in the subtleties of the object. It is a feeling of emptiness (*śūnya*) *and eternal Bliss.*

Continue practicing higher states of *samadhi* with this binaural beats meditation. Binaural beats involve listening to specific audio frequencies designed to enhance relaxation, creativity, and concentration.

This binaural beats meditation will help enhance your experience in meditation and support the continued practice of *samādhi.* (*Scan QR code*)

1.45

sūkṣma-viṣayatvam cāliṅga paryavasānam

The subtle (***sūkṣma***) qualities dissolve into the infinite.

Like a single drop of water falling into the vast ocean and merging seamlessly with the boundless expanse, the meditator's focus enhances and becomes absorbed in increasingly subtle energies that dissolve into the infinite. In this advanced stage of *nirvicārā samādhi*, the meditator transcends the limitations of the senses and the mind.

Journeying beyond the subtle qualities (***sūkṣma***) of thoughts, emotions, and energetic sensations, the realms beyond the physical world are unveiled. Now free from underlying conceptions and memories, we reach a new state of heightened awareness and profound stillness. Pure consciousness, awakens and the yogi deepens their connection to the true essence of Self.

Close your eyes and picture yourself as a drop of water merging into the boundless ocean. With each breath, feel the dissolution of thoughts and emotions as you become increasingly focused on the waves of subtle energy. Descending deeper and dissolving into the vast ocean of consciousness, allow your awareness to expand into the infinite, beyond the boundaries of the senses and the mind. Feel the interconnectedness of your being with the ocean of pure awareness.

Just as a drop merges with the ocean, dissolve into the expansive realm of pure awareness with *Boundless Ocean*, from the Ashtavakra Gita. (*Scan QR code*)

1.46
*tā eva **sa-bījaḥ samādhiḥ***

Each of the previous kinds of samādhi is **sabīja** (with seed or object).

The four stages of *samprajñātaḥ* **samādhi** are with seed or object (**sabīja**). In **sabīja samādhi**, the yogi is fully absorbed in the object of focus, but the potential remains for mental impressions to take hold and grow.

As the yogi immerses in meditation, new thoughts and associations may surface. These impressions can arise from deep layers of the subconscious mind, revealing unresolved emotions, memories, or patterns of conditioning. The advanced yogi observes these arising phenomena without judgment or attachment and allows them to pass through the field of awareness without taking root.

By acknowledging the presence of these mental seeds (**bīja**), we develop a deeper understanding of the interconnected nature of our inner world. This awareness fosters a sense of detachment and objectivity, enabling us to navigate the complexities of the mind with greater clarity and equanimity, without sowing old seeds.

Through continued practice, we gradually refine our ability to meditate while remaining open and receptive to the ever-changing landscape of consciousness. This prepares us for our next state of meditation, **nirbīja samādhi** (without seed), where the mind transcends all objects and fully immerses in the pure essence of being.

1.47

*nirvicāra-vaiśāradye' dhyātma-**prasādaḥ***

When we reach **nirvicāra**-*samādhi*, we encounter the sweet illumination (**prasādaḥ**) of the inner self.

1.48

*ṛtam-bharā tatra **prajñā***

In this state, there is true wisdom (**prajñā**).

1.49

*śrutānumāna-**prajñā**bhyām anya-viṣayā **viśeṣā**rthatvāt*

This true wisdom (**prajñā**) is different from *pramāṇa* and is more focused on the particularities (**viśeṣā**) of the object.

After sitting in the inner silence of *nirvicāra samādhi*, we reach **prasāda**, a profound awakening to our connection with the supreme Self. Within this state of realization lies the gateway to **prajñā**, or deep and transcendent wisdom. **Prajñā** is not to be confused with conventional knowledge, the *pramāṇa* or right knowledge defined in Sūtra 1.7. It is unlike the critical thinking derived from what you see, infer, or learn externally (*pratyaksha-anumāna-agāma*). We can not Google this type of wisdom, find it in a store or attend a lecture to grasp it.

This knowledge can only be known through the *direct experience* of personal meditative practices. By releasing outer distractions, we focus on the deep inner listening that attunes us to the subtle whispers of wisdom within. This wisdom is not our own. It exists beyond definitions from our relative world. Through our exploration, personal questions and inner turbulence naturally find resolution. This cosmic consciousness that flows through the silence changes our being forever.

With the attainment of **prajñā**, the yogi gains the ability to meditate on the subtlest details of objects (**viśeṣā**). This concentrated contemplation opens doors to greater awareness revealing the intricate subtleties of reality.

Begin to sense these intricate subtleties with this Mooji meditation: *The Immensity of Being.* (*Scan QR code*)

1.50

taj-jaḥ saṁskāro 'nya-saṁskāra-pratibandhī

The subconscious impressions generated in *nirvicāra* stop other **saṁskāra** from arising.

1.51

tasyāpi nirodhe sarva-nirodhān nirbījaḥ samādhiḥ

When all impressions dissolve, **nirbīja** (without seed) **samādhi** emerges. Only pure awareness remains without thought or image.

As the clouds of thoughts and all distractions gradually fade away (**sarva-nirodhān**), we enter the highest state of pure awareness. Devoid of the incessant chatter of the mind, it is here, in **nirbīja samādhi**, where we discover the boundless potential of our being.

The yogi now enters *asamprajñāta samādhi*. This state of Enlightenment is pure consciousness without awareness, which is *nirbīja*, free from the seeds of *karma*.

The clear blue sky of our consciousness stretches infinitely before us. The true Self and liberation are now within reach.

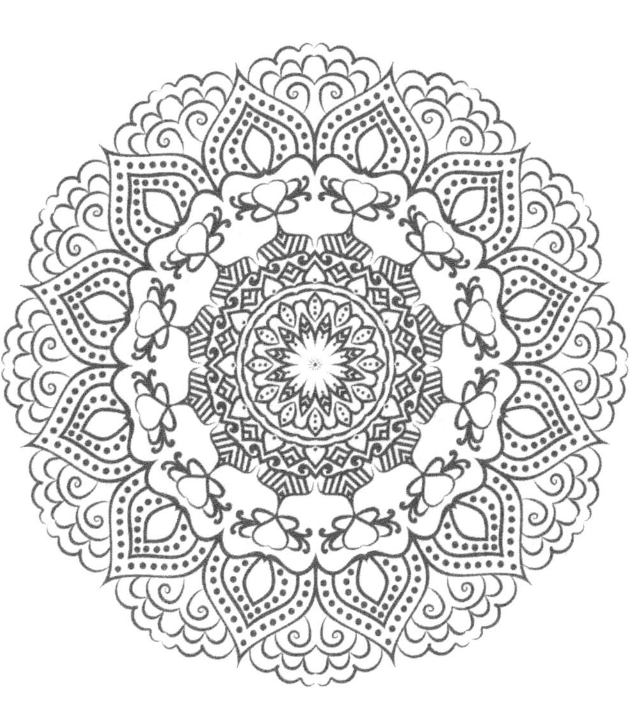

Chapter Two
Sādhana Pāda
The Path to Practice

Sādhana Pāda, translating to "the path of practice", guides us towards the concentration and mental steadiness required to advance our yoga practice. The second Pāda identifies the *kleśas*, the various obstacles that hinder our journey, as well as ways to overcome them. We are also introduced to the first five limbs of *aṣṭāṅga yoga*, the eight-limbed path, also known as *Rāja yoga*. This includes the practical application of ethical and social principles, physical postures, breath control, and the art of drawing inwards.

Let us continue with Pāda Two where ancient wisdom meets modern application.

- Kriyā Yoga: The Yoga of Action (2.1 to 2.2)
- The Five Kleśas: Obstacles Along the Path (2.3 to 2.9)
- Eliminating the Five Kleśas (2.10 to 2.17)
- The Three Guṇas (2.18 to 2.19)
- Puruṣa and Prakṛti (2.20 to 2.25)
- Keen Discernment and Wisdom: Viveka and Prajñā (2.26 to 2.27)
- The First 5 Limbs of the 8 Limb Path (2.28 to 2.56)

2.1 to 2.2
Kriyā Yoga
The Yoga of Action

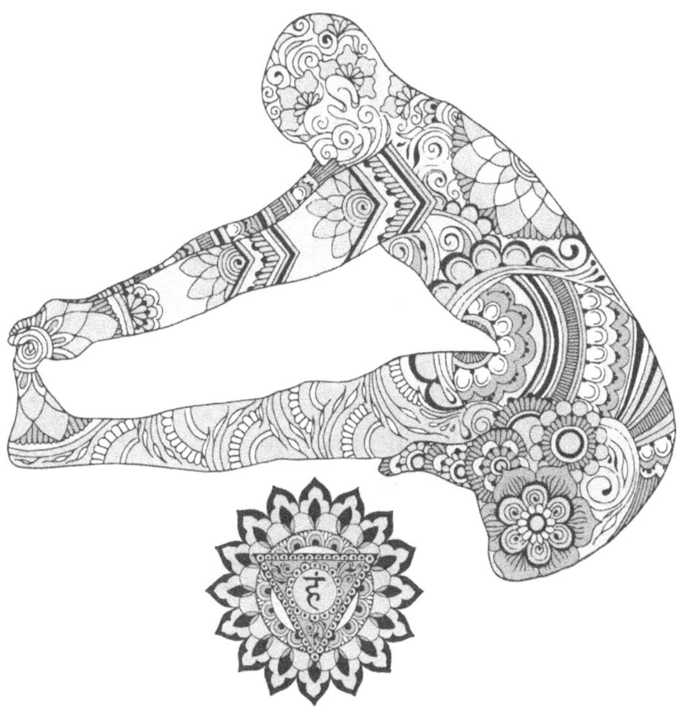

Be courageous in your strength and stay
in the intensity of your practice.

2.1

tapaḥ-svādhyāyeśvara-praṇidhānāni kriyā-yogaḥ

The path to Enlightenment through action is **kriyā yoga**, combining intense practice (**tapas**), self-study, along with the study of yogic texts (**svādhyāya**) and surrender to a higher power (**iśvara-praṇidhānā**).

In Pāda One, we explored approaches to Enlightenment that emphasize the importance of devotion, faith, and patience. Now, Patanjali introduces another path—**kriyā yoga** as a course to Enlightenment through its three pillars:

Tapas, the first pillar, is the unwavering commitment and self-discipline to practice. When we commit with steadfast dedication this serves as the means to purify and transform our being.

Svādhyāya, the second pillar, is the devoted study of yogic texts and engaging in self-reflection. Self-study and pursuing the deeper philosophical aspects of yoga enriches the process of transformation.

Iśvara-praṇidhānā the third pillar, is the surrender to a higher power or the divine flow of life. An essential aspect of *kriyā yoga*, conscious surrender opens the gate to the garden of spiritual awakening.

To further your **svādhyāya** study, here are some helpful resources:

- *Living with the Himalayan Masters by Swami Rama*
- *Light on Life by B.K.S. Iyengar*
- *Think Like a Monk by Jay Shetty*

2.2

*samādhi-bhāvanaarthaḥ **kleśa**-tanū-karaṇārthaś ca*

Through the practice of *kriyā yoga*, we gradually eliminate the five **kleśas** (afflictions), clearing the path to Enlightenment.

While the **kleśas** will be discussed in the following *sūtras*, let us first make note here of the lineage of *Kriyā Yoga*.

This ancient technique traces back to the Upanishads, and although lost for centuries in the Dark Ages, was reintroduced by Lahiri Mahasaya, a renowned yogi of the 19th century. It is believed that Lahiri Mahasaya received personal instruction from Mahavatar Babaji, an immortal yogi, who has guided spiritual seekers throughout the ages.

In 1920, Paramahansa Yogananda arrived in America from his native India and established Self-Realization Fellowship (SRF) to disseminate his *Raja Yoga* teachings, at the heart of which is the sacred *prāṇāyāma* technique of *Kriyā Yoga*. In his groundbreaking book *Autobiography of a Yogi*, as well as in his many other works (including his translation and commentary on the Bhagavad Gita), he writes extensively about the *Kriyā Yoga* science. Today SRF has over 800 temples, ashram centers, and meditation groups worldwide. The services, activities, and offerings of SRF are coordinated by the monastic communities established by Yogananda. Eligible students of the *SRF Lessons* may apply for *Kriyā Yoga* initiation and instruction in this sacred technique by contacting the SRF international headquarters in Los Angeles.

As a part of a daily *Kriyā Yoga* practice, try Yogananda's Energization Exercises, which are designed to enable one to draw cosmic energy consciously into the body, preparing it for meditation. (*Scan QR code*)

(See Additional Resources: Retreat Centers on page 292 for more information on Self-Realization Fellowship initiation.)

2.3 to 2.9
The Five Kleśās
Obstacles Along the Path

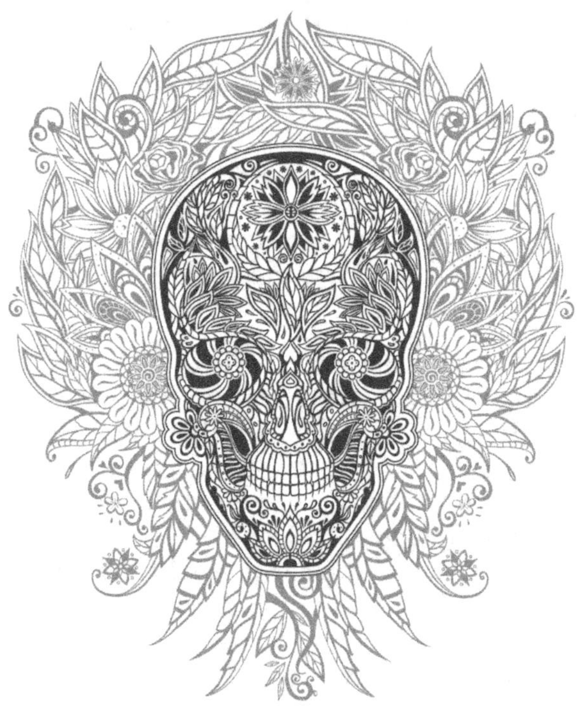

Your trials did not come to punish you but to awaken you.
- Paramahansa Yogananda -

2.3
avidyāsmitā-rāga-dveṣabhiniveśāḥ kleśāḥ

The five **kleśās** are defined as obstacles or miseries that hinder our path to liberation. They are:

1. Unawareness (**avidyā**)
2. Self-centeredness (**asmitā**)
3. Attachment to pleasure (**rāga**)
4. Avoidance of pain (**dveṣa**)
5. Clinging to life or fear of death (**abhiniveśāḥ**)

By practicing *Kriyā Yoga*, we eliminate the five **kleśās** that inhibit our yogic journey. Reflect on the **kleśās** and through self-study (*svādhyāya*) ask yourself:

- **Avidyā**: *How is lacking awareness in my life affecting my well-being?*
- **Asmitā**: *Does my sense of self hinder true happiness?*
- **Rāga**: *What are the things I desire in life? What is the underlying motivation of the things that I desire?*
- **Dveṣa**: *What situations do I avoid or resist? Choose one and make a plan to follow through.*
- **Abhiniveśāḥ**: *What am I afraid to let go of? What daily commitment can I make to myself that will help me overcome this fear?*

Join Shivatman Yoga for a dharma talk on the **kleśās**. (*Scan QR code*)

2.4

Avidyā kṣetram uttareṣām prasupta-tanu-vicchinnodārāṇām

Avidyā, ignorance or lack of knowledge, is the origin from which the other *kleśās* arise, whether in a dormant, weak, intermittent or fully active state.

2.5

*anityāśuci-**duḥkhā**nātmasu nitya-śuci-**sukhā**tma-khyātir **avidyā***

Avidyā arises from mistaking temporary, impure, and painful (**duḥkhā**), things as permanent, pure and pleasurable (**sukhā**).

Avidyā is the root of all suffering and happens when we are blind to our true nature. Due to ignorance, a yogi may mistake suffering for happiness, impermanence for permanence, and the non-self as the Self. It is the first and foremost affliction among the *kleśās* because all the other states of mind arise from it.

When we seek lasting fulfillment by attaching to impermanent experiences, we suffer (**duḥkhā**). **Avidyā** presents in ways such as talking without actively listening, engaging in mindless consumption, or closed-mindedness. Other patterns may surface too including compulsive behaviors such as overeating, excessive use of social media, or other unhealthy habits.

Through dedicated practice of yoga, we free ourselves from the grip of **avidyā**. As we recognize and transcend our detrimental patterns, we awaken a greater understanding of our true Nature.

2.6

Dṛg-darśana-śaktyo ekātmataevāsmitā

Hindering the attainment of *samādhi* is the ego, our self-centeredness (**āsmitā**), which strongly identifies with the material world (*maya*).

Different from our Western conception of ego, **āsmitā** arises not from our arrogance but from our ignorance. **Āsmitā,** the second *kleśā*, refers to our "I-am-that"-ness, the conception of who we think we are that emerges from our attachment to the veiled material world. Our confused sense of self further obscures the truth of our being and reinforces the illusion of separation from our interconnected universe.

Rather than discovering our authentic Self within, our self-importance keeps us focused on seeking identity and fulfillment through outward achievements, material possessions, and external validation. However, by recognizing our unchanging essence (*puruṣa*), we discover where true contentment lies. Centered in awareness, we can choose to transcend the ego and embrace the bliss of our own true Nature.

Reflect on moments when you desired to be the best, look the best, or own the best. These wants are familiar to us all, stemming from societal pressures and personal expectations. Practice sending loving thoughts for others' successes, reevaluating materialistic purchases, and questioning the need for excessive possessions. When we let go of the need for external measures of our worth, we open ourselves to a more authentic and fulfilling experience of life.

For further insight, listen to Anand Ji as he discusses the ego, and *How to Tell When Ego Is Running Your Life (and What to Do Instead)* by Alignment with Veronica. (*Scan QR code*)

2.7
sukhānuśayī rāgaḥ

Rāga is attachment to pleasure (**sukhā**).

When our desire for the repetition of feel-good sensations intensifies, it becomes increasingly challenging to discover the abundance that lies within. **Rāga**, the third *kleśa*, is the clinging and attachment to pleasurable experiences. Pleasure, of course, is not inherently bad and can lead to joy, however, it can also cause suffering.

In our consumer driven society where we are constantly presented with the latest and greatest, it is easy to get caught in the endless cycle of desire. If we "love" someone or something, we need more. We buy a new phone, and a year later, the upgraded version entices us to buy again. We suffer when our attachment to our wants and desires becomes so strong that we find it hard to let them go.

Reflect on **rāga** here:

- *Name a strong attachment to something pleasurable, whether it's a particular experience, possession, or relationship. How does this attachment affect my thoughts, emotions, and actions?*

- *Reflect on the impermanence of pleasurable experiences. How do I typically react when they come to an end?*

- *What attachments do I have to less significant things, like certain foods, clothing, or other material possessions. How do these attachments influence my daily life and decisions?*

If you struggle to let go of attachments, try *Let Go and Let Love* with Anand Ji, on Sattva Connect, and *Yoga Flow To Release Everything, Empty Your Mind... Be Water*, My Friend, Boho Beautiful (26:18) (*Scan QR code*)

2.8
duḥkhānuśayī dveṣaḥ

Dveṣa is avoidance of pain (**duḥkhā**).

It is our natural human tendency to reject things that feel bad and chase after things that feel good. **Dveṣa**, the fourth *kleśā*, is the avoidance of difficult (**duḥkhā**) situations. The development of **dveṣa** (aversion) and **rāga** (desires), of seeing things as good or bad, impacts our wisdom and impedes our personal growth.

We witness **dveṣa** in our lives when we shy away from confronting our fears or challenges. We may choose to avoid situations that make us uncomfortable or anxious, thinking that by doing so, we can maintain a sense of security. However, this avoidance can hinder our personal growth and prevent us from realizing that facing our challenges might lead to greater resilience and well-being. Ironically, sometimes what we avoid could in the end be the most beneficial to our overall growth.

Reflect on aspects of your life that you tend to avoid, such as sharing difficult truths with a friend, attempting a challenging yoga pose, or even mundane tasks like cleaning the house. Create a to-do list and ensure that something you typically avoid is accomplished daily. When we recognize that our challenges do not impact our authentic happiness, we discover there is nothing beyond our reach.

Expand your study of **dveṣa** by listening to this meditation titled *Dealing with Avoidance*. (*Scan QR code*)

2.9

Svarasa-vāhī viduṣo'pi tathārūḍho 'bhiniveśaḥ

Abhiniveśaḥ is clinging to life or fear of death.

Living with a fear of the unknown, especially of the afterlife, prevents us from living a fulfilling life. **Abhiniveśaḥ**, the fifth *kleśa*, is a fear of death that arises from our attachment to the ego and what is familiar. Yoga helps us to let go of our desire to control outcomes and ultimately eliminates this fear. Eventually we learn to see death the same way we see life.

In Eastern traditions, some practice *Maranasati Meditation*, the mindfulness of death. This practice of meditating on death and dying may seem morbid, but it is a powerful way to find peace and acceptance. By recognizing that the wisdom we share and the essence of our being continues on after death, we can find comfort in letting go.

Try answering the question, What will my memorial celebration be like after I die? Describe every detail, including the food and flowers. Leave this description of your desires with your will, letting go of the fear of death and embracing the impermanence of life.

Incorporating savāsana, or corpse pose, into your yoga practice for at least five minutes at the end of each class can also help with this process. Visualize yourself merging with divine consciousness and feel the release that comes from awakening to this infinite state of being.

Uncover more insight with, *Guided Death Meditation to Live More* (Maranasati), by The Downward Doug. (*Scan QR code*)

2.10 to 2.17
Eliminating the Five Kleśās

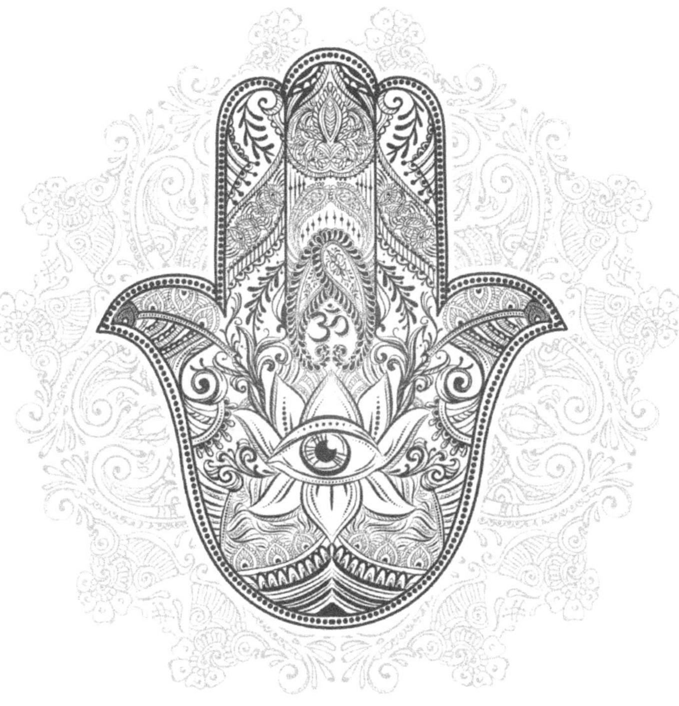

In the pursuit of knowledge, every day something is added.
In the practice of the Tao, everyday something is dropped.
- Laozi -

2.10

Te pratiprasava-heyāḥ sūkṣmāḥ

With practice, one dissolves the subtle (**sūkṣmāḥ**) seeds of the *kleśas*.

2.11

Dhyāna-heyās tad-vṛttayaḥ

These fluctuations of the mind (**vṛittis**) are eliminated through meditation (**dhyāna**).

As we continue on our yogic journey we become *Witnesses* of our inner being and the world around us. From our *witness* state, we access the wisdom to recognize the inner impurities of the *kleśas* before they affect our actions. Eventually, we open the door to releasing their hold on us all together.

As our practice deepens, our awareness expands, desires diminish, pain is released, and the tight hold of worldly concerns eases. The power of the *kleśas* begins to lose its grasp on our consciousness. When we enter the highest state of spiritual involution in deep meditation, the *kleśas* ultimately dissolve.

Imagine yourself in deep meditation and becoming angry, afraid, or craving. This is impossible. The more we cultivate a regular meditation practice, the more our true nature of calmness and stability emerges.

Quiet the mind with this *5 Minute Mindfulness Meditation* by Sherri Lukac and Red House Wellness. (*Scan QR code*)

2.12

Kleśa-mūlaḥ karmāśayo dṛṣṭādṛṣṭ a-janma-vedanīyaḥ

The **Kleśa-mūlaḥ** are the root of the **karmāśayo**, an accumulation of impressions that influence present and future experiences.

Kleśa-mūlaḥ, the roots of afflictions, can be compared to weeds that have taken root in the garden of our consciousness. These mental distortions, like invasive plants, disrupt the harmony of our inner landscape and overshadow the delicate flowers of our true nature.

Just as a skilled gardener tends to their garden, we can weed our **kleśas**. Through diligent practice, we acquire the ability to recognize the buds of our deep-seated afflictions as well as the **karmāśayo**, the accumulation of these impressions and experiences that source our suffering. By pulling them from their roots, we cultivate a fertile ground to nourish inner growth.

This garden of **kleśa-mūlaḥ** impedes our ability to make positive decisions and overcome obstacles. When we are shaped by painful hardships such as childhood trauma or challenging relationships, detaching from the **kleśas** can be especially difficult. Through consistent practice, we become less affected by the wounds and scars we carry and gradually alleviate our suffering.

This Insight Timer meditation by Daniel Roquéo, *Egoic Mantra* will guide you through the process of becoming aware of and releasing the two core beliefs of the ego: *"I Am Not Enough"* and *"There Is Not Enough."* (*Scan QR code*)

2.13

*sati **mūle** tad-vipāko jāty-āyur-bhogāḥ*

The root (***mūle***) of our actions (*karma*) is based on collective *saṁskāras*

Our storehouse of actions (*karmāśayo*) is the root (***mūle***) of deeply ingrained impressions that lead to certain cultural or societal behaviors. Like a tree with roots hidden beneath the soil, our karmic patterns will continue to produce the fruits of our actions until we address their underlying origins. Cutting down the tree is insufficient; we must dig deeper and destroy the roots themselves.

Yoga helps us to alter our physical and emotional responses to these impressions (*saṁskāras*). Instead of trying to push or pray away our feelings, in meditation we gradually move through a process of releasing them. The more often we show up for ourselves, the more we peel away the layers of our *saṁskāras*, like peeling away the layers of an onion. The more we remain present, the more we let go.

Consider this practice for burning *saṁskāras* metaphorically:

Find a quiet and comfortable space. Light a candle or create a small bonfire in a safe place, symbolizing the fire of transformation. Take a few deep breaths to center yourself. Bring to mind a lingering saṁskāra. Write down a few words that represent this saṁskāra on a small piece of paper.

Hold the intention that you are ready to transform this saṁskāra. Offer this piece of paper to the flame, watching it burn and disintegrate into ash. As it transforms, visualize the negative impression turning into light, releasing you from its grip. Sit in stillness for a few moments, feeling the release and the newfound freedom within.

Try this meditation *Permission to Let Go* by The Mindful Movement to release suppressed emotions. (*Scan QR code*)

2.14

*Te hlāda-paritāpa-phalāḥ **puṇyāpuṇya**-hetutvāt.*

The fruits of our actions can be pleasurable (**puṇyā**) or painful (**āpuṇya**).

According to the Law of Attraction, the energy we put out into the world attracts like experiences. When we cultivate positive intentions, those rooted in love, compassion, and kindness, we create a ripple effect that draws forth joy and harmony. These virtuous actions generate **puṇyā**, or joyful outcomes, which contribute to our overall well-being and the well-being of those around us.

Conversely, when our actions are driven by negativity, selfishness, or harmful intentions, we set in motion a chain of events that lead to pain, suffering, and discord. These harmful actions result in **āpuṇya**, or negative outcomes, which bring about disharmony and further perpetuate the cycle of suffering.

To navigate this intricate web of cause and effect, it is essential to make conscious choices rooted in love (*prema*). By choosing love over fear, love over disappointment, love over anger, and love over jealousy, we learn to live in a place of love in every moment, empowering us to make wiser decisions and align with our highest values.

Remember to Choose Love! By Great Meditation. (*Scan QR code*)

2.15

*Pariṇāma-tāpa-saṁskāra-duḥkhair guṇa-vṛtti-virodhāc
ca **duḥkham** eva sarvaṁ **vivekinaḥ***

Those with discrimination (**viveka**) recognize that life is suffering as a result of inevitable hardships (**duhka**), shifts in energy (**guṇas**) and impressions (**saṁskāras**) arising from the *citta-vṛttis*.

In the shadow of *avidyā*, our vision may be clouded, and we may fail to recognize the fundamental truth that everything is suffering. This philosophical principle rooted in Mahayana Buddhism teaches that all aspects of existence are perfused with suffering, including even the seeming joy of virtuous deeds.

When attention is trapped in the material world, we gravitate towards enjoyment (*rāga*) and avoid pain (*dveṣa*). This focus on the external, we've seen, leads to suffering. Those who incessantly seek sources of joy outside themselves, rather than turning inward, miss genuine contentment. This is not to say that finding joy outside of ourselves is inherently bad, however, true and lasting contentment is not found soley in external pursuits.

The **vivekina**, equipped with discrimination and discernment, directs attention inward to seek true wisdom, joy, and connection with the essence of Self. Knowing that infinite Bliss–*ānanda*–is not discovered in the busyness of the outer world, the **vivekina** quietly explores and finds answers from within.

Release negative energy and end suffering with the following meditation by davidji. (*Scan QR code*)

2.16

*Heyaṁ **duḥkha**m anāgatam*

Pain and suffering (**dukha**), which is yet to come, can be avoided.

2.17

Draṣṭr-dṛśyayoḥ saṁyogo heya-hetuḥ

Suffering caused by the Seer's (**draṣṭr**) attachment to the material world (**dṛśya**) can be avoided.

Our perception affects our experiences. When we identify with the material world (*dṛśya*), we become attached to its fleeting pleasures and inevitably experience pain. We have the choice, however, not to suffer. By nurturing our inner universe through a dedicated practice, we detach from worldly desires and experience lasting serenity.

As we learned in Pāda One, consistency is the key to avoid suffering and to allow our inner space to unfold. Try different styles of yoga and meditation to find what resonates with you most, and commit to a daily practice. Remember, the journey is not about perfection, but the effort and consistency put forth. With time and practice, the benefits will become apparent as the *kleśas* dissolve.

Let go of past suffering with *Rewrite the Past* on *Sattvaconnect.com*.
(*Scan QR code*)

2.18 to 2.19
The Three Gunas

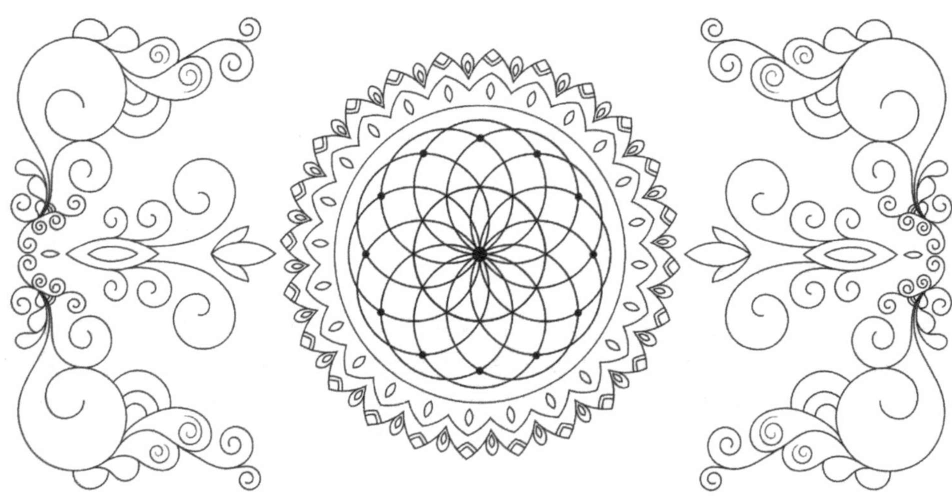

He who sees inaction in action and who sees action in inaction,
he is the one endowed with wisdom among human beings.
He is joined in yoga, a performer of complete action.

- Bhagavad Gita Ch. 4 V.18 -

2.18

*Prakāśa-kriyā-sthiti-śīlaṁ bhūtendriyātmakaṁ
bhogāpavargārthaṁ **dṛśyam***

All things in the Universe that are known (**dṛśya**) possess a nature of illumination (**prakāśa**), activity (**kriyā**), and inertia (**sthiti**), composed of the elements and senses, and exists for the purpose of either liberation or experience (**bhogā**).

Sūtra 1.16 teaches that *samādhi* leads to freedom from the *guṇas*. Now we learn more about how the *guṇas*, the subtle underlying forces of energy, are the means of experiencing life (**bhogā**) and liberation (*kaivalya*).

Everything that is known and experienced (**dṛśya**) possesses three energies: **prakāśa** (illuminated energy), **kriyā** (active energy) and **sthiti** (energy that is still). The energetic nature of our lives correlates with the properties of the underlying *guṇas*: **prakāśa** with *sattva*, **kriyā** with *rajas*, and **sthiti** *with tamas.*

By drawing our awareness to the present moment, we can observe and regulate our energy states, settling into the harmonious space between effort and surrender. When we find ourselves in a stressful state, we can pause and find balance using the tools of yoga. Having a sense of humor, too, can help to change our state of being.

Commit to a day of observing your energy. Witness how often you are in a state of rajas (energetic), tamas (lethargic), or sattva (peaceful and balanced). Can you recognize when your authentic Self has taken a back seat and when the guṇas have become your driver? At this very moment, pause and check in with your energetic state. What do you notice and what steps can you take to be more mindful of how you use your energy?

2.19

Viśeṣāviśeṣaliṅga-mātrāliṅgāni guṇa-parvāṇi.

The stages of the **guṇas** pass through the four states of existence: gross, subtle, primal, and unmanifest.

As we self unfold, we explore the intricate dance of the four stages of energy—**viśeṣā** (the particularized), **aviśeṣa** (the unparticularized), **liṅga** (the concrete), and **aliṅga** (unmanifested)—and how these states shape our perception of reality.

Viśeṣā forms the foundation of our world, encompassing the tangible elements of *prakṛti*: earth, water, fire, air, and ether. The subtle nuances of **aviśeṣa** are the unparticularized qualities emerging from the individual self (*ahaṁkāra*). These are the vibrations of sound, touch, sight, taste, and smell. **Liṅga**, or *manas*, unfolds directly from the intellect and logic that connects us to the vast intelligence within. From subtler realms is **aliṅgā**, the unmanifested—the potential energy of *prakṛti* waiting to unfurl.

As a yogi, we continually evolve and move into more subtle states of existence. In the process of evolution, the movement is from subtle to gross. In yoga, however, we practice the process of involution—moving from gross to subtle.

Meditate on the subtler states of being by practicing cellular breathing. Imagine oxygen passing through the boundaries of one cell as carbon dioxide and waste exit. As you continue to breath, experience the subtle waves of movement and let your awareness expand to multiple cells within. Feel the vibrant energy circulating with each breath.

Continue with *Cellular Breathing in the Bones* by Mark Taylor. (*Scan QR code*)

2.20 to 2.25
Puruṣa and Prakṛti

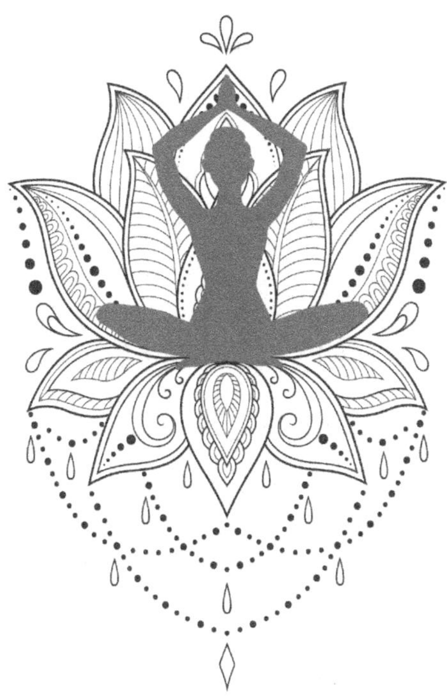

There is the mud, and there is the lotus that grows out of the mud.
We need the mud in order to make the lotus.

- Thich Nhat Hanh -

2.20

Draṣṭā dṛśi-mātraḥ śuddho 'pi pratyayānupaśyaḥ

The Seer (**draṣṭā**) is pure consciousness, although it appears to see through mental concepts (**pratyayā**).

Draṣṭā, the Seer, is our inner spirit that perceives the world through the lens of the mind. It is the spark of pure consciousness within each of us known as *ātman*. Though the Seer is inherently pure, *ātman* observes our world through the filter of mental constructs or conceptions (**pratyayā**) that arise in the mind.

The *Guṇa Sūtras* remind us that everything in the universe, including ourselves, is made up of energy vibrating at different frequencies. Even the densest forms of matter are intricate webs of vibration. The sun, a tree, a towering building, the mat you sit upon–everything is an expression of the pure consciousness that underlies it. Contemplating this metaphysical truth opens the doorway to expanding our awareness.

When we meditate on this reality, we recognize that the essence of consciousness that resides within us also resides within every individual. This realization frees us from the illusion of separation, awakening our understanding of the interconnectedness of humanity. As this truth begins to guide our actions and interactions, we foster empathy, compassion, and a deep appreciation for the interwoven fabric of existence.

Explore this concept with Ram Das on Spotify called *Awareness. (Scan QR code)*

2.21
*Tad-**artha** eva dṛśyasyātmā*

That which is seen exists solely for the purpose of spiritual essence (*ātmā*).

Imagine the essence of our **ātmān** like a beautiful lotus flower, its petals gracefully unfurling upon the surface of a murky pond. The lotus symbolizes the **ātmān**, the spark of *puruṣa* within each of us. The pond's muddy depths represent the material world, *prakṛti*, where our senses plunge into a constant whirlwind of experiences.

In yoga philosophy, the material world (*prakṛti*)—the mud—exists to be experienced by the lotus, our **ātmān**, our inner spark of *puruṣa*. Like the lotus emerging from the mud, the purpose of the seen, the external world, is to serve and inform the Seer. Despite the challenges and impurities surrounding it, the *ātmān* remains pure and untouched by the material world. With diligent practice, we disentangle the Seer from the captivating illusions of the seen.

As we delve deeper into meditation and self-reflection, the lotus of our true nature blossoms, indifferent to the muddiness of external distractions. The purpose of all that which is seen becomes clear—it's here to help us recognize, embrace and experience our inherent *dharma*, our life's purpose, and the true nature of our being. In the light of our authentic Self, we unearth the ultimate freedom of divine Bliss.

Embrace the metaphor of the lotus flower with this meditation by Braydon Mackenzie. (*Scan QR code*)

2.22

kṛtārtham prati naṣṭam apy anaṣṭam tad-anya-sādhāraṇatvāt

Though the seen (*dṛśya*) may cease once its purpose is fulfilled, the Seer (*ātma*) is Infinite.

As our lotus flower unfurls, we release the tight grip of the *kleśas* and discover our untethered and boundless nature.

When our attachment to the mortal self loosens, we are drawn towards the infinite Self within—the pure awareness that is not subject to gain or loss. Here, we discover our true essence, the radiant lotus—the eternal Seer (*ātma*). We bask in the wholeness that transcends fleeting achievements and experience contentment from the inside out, rather than the outside in.

In this illuminated state of existence, the ordinary becomes extraordinary, and joy is found in the simplest of things—a bird's song, a heartfelt conversation, or savoring each bite of a sweet dessert. This heightened awareness of the present moment, unburdened from our attachment to external outcomes, allows us to embrace life's beauty in its purest form. In the eternal dance of existence, the Seer remains as the ever-present Witness to the fleeting scenes of the seen.

Embrace the essence of your radiant Self by repeating the *padma* or lotus flower mantra. (*Scan QR code*)

Om mani padme hum, Om mani padme hum, Om mani padme hum.

Awaken to the jewel of the radiant lotus.

2.23

Svas-vāmi-śaktyoḥ **svarūpo***palabdhi-hetuḥ* **saṁyogaḥ***.*

The union (**saṁyogaḥ**) between the seen and the Seer is the basis [for understanding that] which is eternal from that which is not.

2.24

Tasya hetur **avidyā**

The [suffering] caused by this union stems from ignorance (**avidyā**).

2.25

Tad-abhāvāt **saṁyogā***bhāvo hānaṁ tad-dṛśeḥ* **kaivalyam**

When ignorance (**avidyā**) is removed, the Seer rests in their own true Self (**svarūpe**) and finds Absolute Freedom (**kaivalya**).

When we settle into the infinite joy that resides within, we unearth the ultimate truth: amidst the interconnectedness of everything in our Universe, a clear distinction remains between *puruṣa* (the Seer) and *prakṛti* (the seen).

By nurturing spiritual awareness, we begin to understand that everything that exists in our world is illuminated by the same underlying spark of consciousness. As we dissolve our ignorance (**avidyā**) through the process of self-inquiry and develop greater awareness, the truth of our reality is revealed to us. The removal of our ignorance leads to the recognition of the Seer—the radiant lotus, our innermost Self—and the realization of *kaivalya*, the state of absolute Freedom.

Today, be the Witness, the Watcher and the Experiencer. When you find yourself having a challenging day or feeling overwhelmed with the murkiness of life, take pause and bring awareness to atha, the present moment. Instead of identifying with your citta-vṛttis, your states of mind, return to your inherent nature. Inquire within and ask yourself, "Who is unhappy? Who is having a bad day? Who is sad?" Observe life as it unfolds around you. Do not react, do not judge, just observe.

Find your mindful seat and sit upon your lily pad. Whether you are feeling happy, sad, positive, or negative, sit with your emotions without judgment, resistance, or attachment, and meditate on them with a sense of curiosity. Label them as passing experiences, not aspects of yourself that define your identity. Just as clouds come and go in the sky, allow the impermanent emotions and thoughts to arise and subside in your field of consciousness.

By observing them with detached awareness, we gradually dissolve their grip and recognize the essence of who we truly are—the blossoming lotus flower.

2.26 to 2.27
Keen Discernment and Wisdom
Viveka and Prajñā

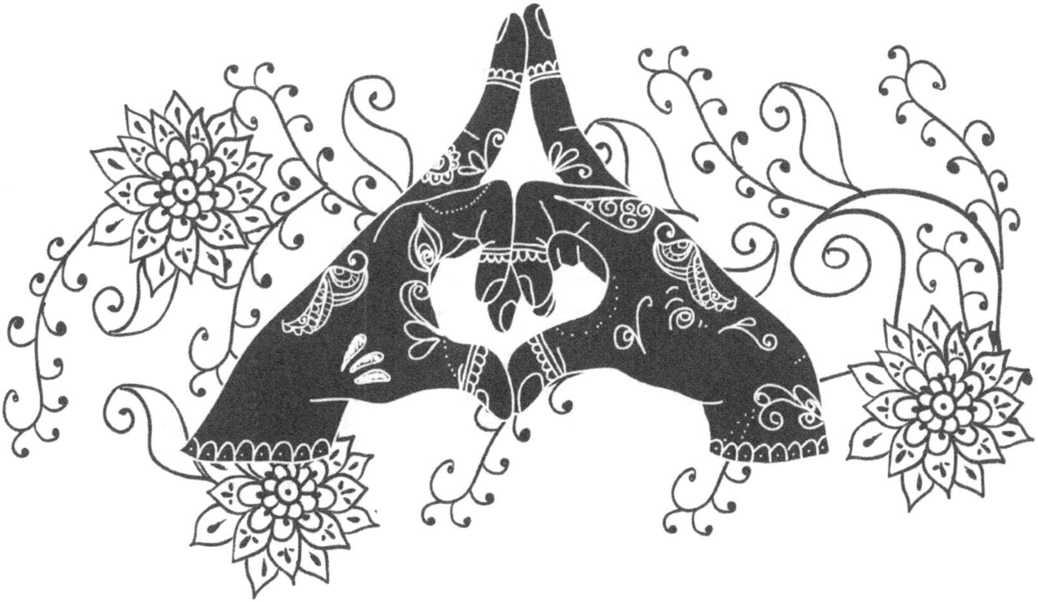

Verily, nothing else in the world is as sanctifying as wisdom.
In due course of time, the devotee who is successful in yoga
will spontaneously realize this within his Self.
- The Bhagavad Gita Ch IV:V.38 -

2.26
Viveka-khyātir aviplavā hānopāyaḥ

Keen discernment (**viveka**) destroys ignorance (*avidya*).

Through consistent practice, we access **viveka**, or discriminative discernment, which requires deep self-awareness and self-reflection. This nurtures our ability to navigate life's challenges with clear insight and make choices aligned with our highest purpose.

In our physical practice, **viveka** allows us to approach poses mindfully and in a way that considers our readiness. By approaching intensity from a place of conscious awareness, and making choices that stretch our boundaries but respect our limits, our practice flourishes. Disciplines that explore the many aspects and layers of ourselves, include Bhakti yoga for devotion, meditation for introspection, *prānāyāma* for breath control, and *āsana* to connect with the body. Through the integration of discernment, we feel and experience *prajñā*—the guiding wisdom that facilitates the balance between effort and surrender leading to ease both on and off the mat.

Explore different levels of intensity in your yoga practice and allow *viveka* to guide you. Here are three practices of varying levels (*Scan QR code*):

Silent Yin Yoga, The Bare Female
Intermediate / *Shoulders and Upper Back* with Yoga Awakening
Advanced / Intermediate Yoga Flow with Boho Beautiful

2.27

*Tasya saptadhā prānta-bhūmiḥ **prajñā**.*

When the yogi develops wisdom (**prajñā**) there are seven insights gained.

Through the development of discernment, wisdom emerges. The wisdom described as **prajñā** is not intellectual knowledge, or critical thinking. It is a deeper knowing that arises through direct experience. Empowered with **prajñā**, we see through illusions and gain an understanding of the true essence of our existence.

Though not listed in the *sūtra* itself, the seven insights gained are taught by commentators from Vyāsa to Swami Satchidananda. With **prajñā** the yogi now knows:

1) Where happiness lies and what needs to be avoided to maintain *sattva*.

2) The *kleśas* can be eradicated.

3) Less is more.

4) An unlimited source of knowledge exists within.

5) How to end sorrow and live in a state of peace.

6) How to maintain the harmonious and balanced energy of the *guṇas*.

7) The true Self is independent of the material world.

Deep unfoldment of wisdom requires persistent practice and unwavering dedication, but the attainment of **prajñā** is available to all. Keep progressing along your journey towards all seven insights.

2.28 to 2.56
The First 5 Limbs of the 8 Limb Path
Yamas-Niyamas-Āsana-Prāṇāyāma-Pratyāhāra

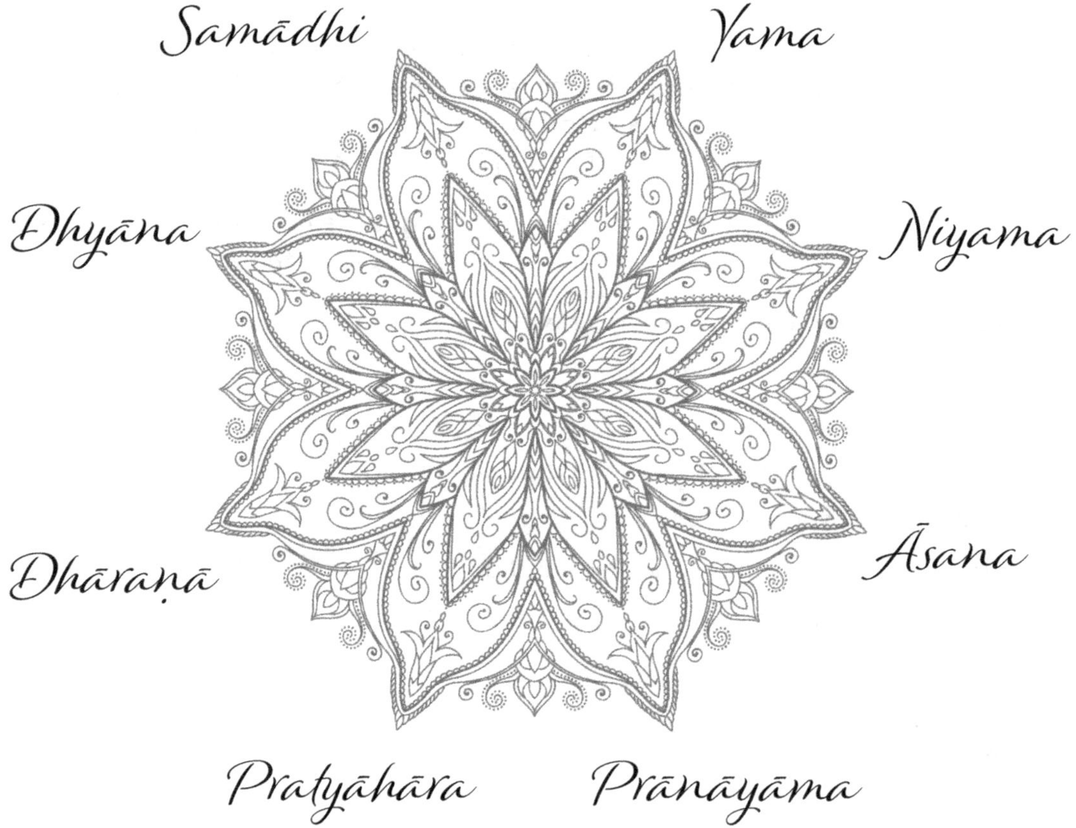

2.28

*Yogāṅgānuṣṭhānād aśuddhi- kṣaye **jñāna**-dīptir- ā **viveka**-khyāteḥ.*

Diligently practice the limbs (***āṅgā***) of **yoga,** and the afflictions of life (*kleśas*) will gradually diminish, leading to the emergence of profound knowledge (***jñāna***) and insight (***viveka***).

Patanjali has been guiding us on our journey of self-discovery thus far by unveiling the *kleśas* that hinder our progress and ways to overcome them. Now, a direct route to freedom is introduced—*aṣṭāṅga* and the *Rāja Yoga path*.

Rāja Yoga, the royal path, is the comprehensive framework of the eight limbs (***āṅgā***) of yoga. Different from the earlier yoga systems of *Bhakti*, *Jñāna*, and *Karma*, the eight limbs touch upon all aspects of our being and promise the reward of keen insight (***viveka***) and divine knowledge (***jñāna***).

It is important to note that the term *aṣṭāṅga* in this context should not be confused with Pattabhi Jois's Ashtanga Yoga, which refers to a specific practice involving several series of repeated and perfected sequences. Pattabhi Jois introduced his Ashtanga Yoga system to the United States in the 1970s. (*Scan QR code*)

To commence our study of the 8 limbs let's begin with a sun salutation practice. Consider waking up to this practice every morning. (*Scan QR code*)

2.29

Yama-niyamāsana-prāṇāyāma-pratyāhāra-dhāraṇā-dhyāna-samādhayo 'ṣṭāv aṅgāni

Patanjali presents the eight limbs (**aṅgā**) of yoga.

1. **Yamas**: Societal or Moral Responsibilities that concern our relationship with ourselves and others.
   - **Ahimsā** – Non-harming
   - **Satyā** – Truthfulness
   - **Asteya** – Non-stealing
   - **Brahmacaryā** – Conservation of energy
   - **Āparigrahā** – Letting go

2. **Niyamas**: Personal duties that nurture our individual growth and well-being.
   - **Śauca** – Self-purifications
   - **Saṁtoṣa** – Contentment
   - **Tapas** – Disciplines
   - **Svādyāya** – Self-study and study of scriptures
   - **Īśvara praṇidhāna** – Surrender to a higher power

3. **Āsana** – Physical practice

4. **Prāṇāyāma** – Controlled breathing techniques

5. **Pratyāhāra** – Letting go of sensory distractions / sensory withdrawal

6. **Dhāraṇā** – Concentration

7. **Dhyāna** – Meditation

8. **Samādhi** – Enlightenment / Meditative Absorption

2.30

Ahiṁsā-satyāsteya-brahmacaryāparigrahā yamāḥ

The **yamas** are broken down into 5 categories: non-harming, truthfulness, non-stealing, non-excess and letting go.

2.31

*Jāti-deśa-kāla-samayānavacchinnāḥ **sārva-bhaumā mahā-vratam.***

The *yamas* are great vows (**mahā-vrata**) made to oneself and to others. They are universal (**sārva-bhaumā**), and no account is given to class, place, time or circumstance.

1. ***Ahiṁsa*** - Non-harming to self or others
2. ***Satyā*** - Truthfulness
3. ***Asteya*** - Non-stealing
4. ***Brahmacaryā*** - Non-excess, self-control
5. ***Āparigrahā*** - Non-greed

Prescribed as a universal code of morality, the *yamas* are the deep promises we make with the world and with ourselves to practice non-harming, honesty, taking less, moderation, and wanting less. By honoring these great vows, we act from our commitment to universal wisdom and love in all situations.

The *yamas* also mark the beginning of a bigger pledge that we make with ourselves—to manifest and share our authentic spirit in every facet of life.

2.32

Śauca-saṁtoṣa-tapaḥ-svādhyāyeśvara-praṇidhānāni niyamāḥ

The **niyamās**, daily observances or habits, include self-purification, contentment, discipline, self-study, and surrender.

The **niyamās** are broken down into five categories.

1. **Śauca** – Purification of mind, body, and speech

2. **Saṁtoṣa** – Contentment within and without

3. **Tapas** – Self-discipline and endurance

4. **Svādhyāya** – Self-study and self-reflection

5. **Iśvara praṇidhānā** – Surrendering to a higher power or divine consciousness

After the great vows of the *yamas*, we progress to the **niyamās**, the second limb. The **niyamās,** translated as observances, are the personal behaviors and restraints that shape our conduct from the inside out. Building awareness around our individual behaviors allows us to make meaningful changes in our daily lives. By practicing the **niyamās**, we engage in true acts of self-improvement. These self-care practices not only enhance our personal wellness, but also influence our daily actions and habits.

Sūtras 2.40-2.45 will discuss and expand upon the **niyamās**.

2.33 to 2.39
The 1st Limb of the 8 Limb Path

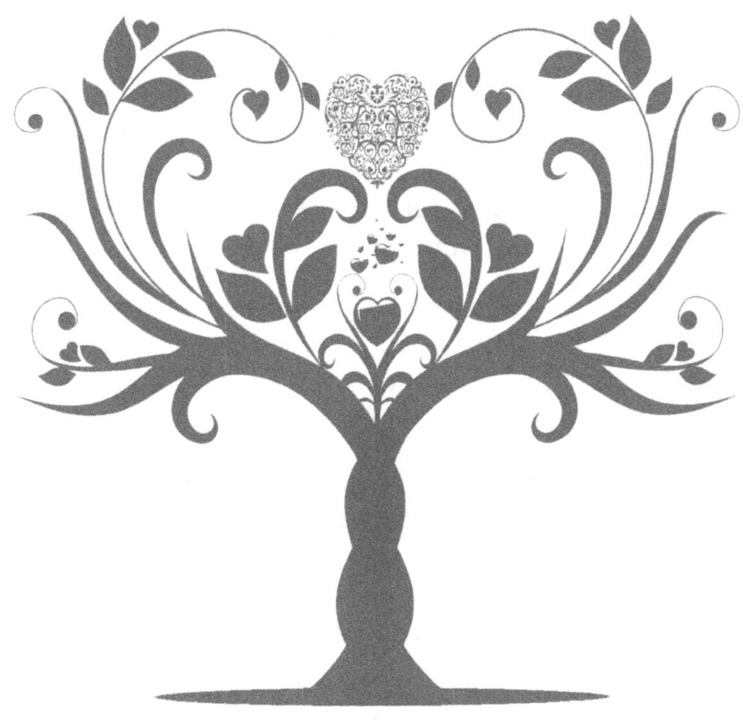

The Yamas
Great Vows

2.33

*Vitarka-bādhane **pratipakṣa-bhāvanam***

When disturbed by negative thoughts, turn towards positive ones. This is the practice of **pratipakṣa bhāvanam**, the cultivation of opposites.

In every moment we are presented with a choice: to dwell on our fears and worries or to consciously refocus on the good in our lives. This *sūtra* emphasizes the power of embracing the principle of the first *yama*, *ahimsā*. By shifting our mindset from negative to positive with **pratipakṣa bhāvanam**, we nurture a compassionate environment that supports our mental and emotional well-being.

Gratitude is an impactful tool for cultivating a positive mindset. Take a few moments each day to reflect on the blessings in your life, fostering an attitude of appreciation. Observe how this practice nurtures contentment by shifting your focus towards the uplifting and joyful aspects of your existence.

*Try actively putting **pratipakṣa bhāvanam** into practice with this exercise. Transform each negative thought into three positive ones, and gradually expand the scope over time. Best-selling author Jay Shetty suggests in his book Think Like a Monk that, to unlock the full potential of this practice, we should aim to generate ten positive thoughts for each negative one. The goals you set are up to you.*

Here is a beautiful gratitude practice with Mindful Movement called *5 Minute Guided Meditation for Gratitude*. (*Scan QR code*)

2.34

*Vitarkā hiṁsādayaḥ kṛta-kāritānumoditā lobha-krodha-moha-pūrvakā mṛdu madhyādhimātrā **duḥkhā**jñānānanta-phalā iti**pratipakṣabhāvanam**.*

Negative thoughts and words are a form of violence (***vitarkā hiṁsā***). They may be triggered by greed, anger, and delusion of varying intensity.

Our words do more than tell a story, they *create one*. When we gossip or judge, we manifest negativity and send pain (***duḥkhā***) into the world. When our practice is steady and without pause we release this harmful energy and create new and compassionate thoughts. Through reflection and the practice of ***pratipakṣa bhāvanam***, we end the cycle of harm and suffering.

*Whether speaking ill of others or engaging in negative self-talk, take a moment to recognize the **hiṁsā** energy that is gathering like a dark cloud. Before harm rains down, take pause to spot, feel, and swap. Spot your own greed, anger, and delusion. Feel this energy in your body. Then swap this negativity with a kind thought or action, allowing the storm within to pass. Internally repeat the mantra, "My feelings are not serving me physically and mentally," and smile in the clear, open space of self-awareness.*

By creating loving thoughts towards others and ourselves, we take orbit in a sphere of kindness, gratitude, and empathy. When you observe ***vitarkā hiṁsā***, make the choice to practice ***pratipakṣa bhāvanam***.

This guided meditation focuses on the principle of ***ahiṁsā*** by 365 Days of Meditation. (*Scan QR code*)

2.35

Ahiṁsā pratiṣṭhāyām tat samnidhau vaira tyāgaḥ.

All threats and hostilities are abandoned by one truly established in the practice of nonviolence (**ahiṁsā**).

Envision a world in which every child learns the principles of yoga, embracing **ahiṁsā** as a way of life. In this enlightened future, the great vow we take to practice non-harming transforms us, and holds the power to transform our universe.

In *sūtra* 2.33 we learned that violence extends to actions beyond physical harm. Breaking **ahiṁsā** includes verbal aggression, mental abuse, and any mistreatment inflicted upon others or ourselves. Through meditation we deepen our understanding of the many forms of violence, and gradually free ourselves from all conflict.

By embodying *ahiṁsā* in all aspects of our existence, our deeply rooted commitment builds a circle of peace where hostilities naturally fade away and love prevails. Holding steadfast to this pledge of non-violence, what we radiate out reflects back to us.

Practice this meditation daily, creating universal harmony and seeing the reflection of ourselves in others. This mindfulness meditation has roots in the *metta* of Buddhism:

> *May 'I' be happy, free from pain and suffering, peaceful, and full of bliss.*
>
> *May 'You' be happy, free from pain and suffering, peaceful, and full of bliss.*
>
> *May 'We' be happy, free from pain and suffering, peaceful, and full of bliss.*

 Continue with the following loving-kindness meditation. (*Scan QR code*)

2.36

Satya pratiṣṭhāyām kriyāphalāśrayatvam.

Through honesty and truthfulness (**satya**), we reap the fruit of our actions.

Satya is honesty. The second *niyama* reflects not only telling the truth when it leads to no harm, but also being true to oneself. By being honest with ourselves and living with integrity, our *karma* yields personal abundance guiding our progression on the path.

Satya encompasses not only expressing our truth with kindness and compassion, but also listening to the truth of others, even when it's uncomfortable or challenging. By remaining rooted in love while acknowledging another person's perspective and feelings, we create space to heal and grow in and beyond our relationships.

Reflect on the following questions:

- *Are my relationships with friends and family members true to my life's ideals?*
- *Am I living my truth through my work?*
- *Do I engage in activities that are consistent with my virtues and values?*
- *Do I listen to the truth of others, even when it is uncomfortable or challenging?*

On the mat, we can support honest communication by practicing throat openers. Poses like puppy dog pose (*anahatāsana*) and fish pose (*matsyāsana*) stretch our voices and our hearts in ways that nurture healthy self-expression.

We can also use the mantra: *"I follow and speak my truth. I listen to the truth of others,"* reminding us of the importance of both speaking and hearing the truth.

2.37

*Asteya*pratiṣṭhāyām sarvaratnopasthānam.

Asteya (*non-stealing*) brings an abundance of treasures.

Asteya is the practice of being content with what is ours. The third *yama*, non-stealing, cultivates a mindset of abundance and fulfillment rather than of scarcity or greed.

Asteya teaches us that when we let go of excessive desire and refrain from taking what belongs to others, we are rewarded with inner abundance. This concept extends beyond the theft of material goods and includes stealing others time, energy, and ideas. When we practice **asteya**, we become established in trust and respect that adds a kaleidoscope of richness to our lives.

To practice **asteya**, ask yourself:

- Am I taking what belongs to others?
- Am I giving credit where credit is due?
- Am I keeping my promises and respecting other people's time?
- Am I cultivating a sense of gratitude and contentment in my life?

On the mat, practice poses that cultivate strength and stability, such as Warrior I and II (*Vīrabhadrāsana* I and II). Off the mat, we can practice generosity and giving to others *without expecting anything in return*.

Explore **asteya** with this *prāṇāyāma* and sound vibrations meditation with Sarah Margaret on Insight Timer. (*Scan QR code*)

2.38

Brahmacarya pratiṣṭhāyām vīryalābhaḥ.

*By practicing **brahmacarya** one attains vitality and energy (**vīrya**).*

Brahmacarya, translates as celibacy, but reflects a restraint that extends beyond sexual abstinence. The fourth *yama* is the moderation and wise use of our energy in all areas of life, including in our actions and thoughts. When we excessively use energy, whether it be on our mats, in our conversations, or in any other aspect of our lives, it drains our life force and keeps us from a harmonious and balanced existence.

Through the practice of **brahmacarya**, we learn to balance and manage our energy that allows our inner light to remain charged from morning until night. Empowered by our steady flow of vitality, our creativity and passions thrive.

Ask yourself:

- *What in life drains my energy? Is it over-exercising, excessive spending, sexual activity, toxic relationships, overeating or overwork?*
- *In this very moment, what is the best use of my energy, whether it be on the yoga mat, communicating with someone, or transforming negative thoughts?*

On the mat, practice *prānāyāma* exercises such as *nāḍī shodhana* (alternate nostril breathing) to balance the flow of energy in the body. Practice grounding yoga poses such as *tadasana* (mountain pose) and *balasana* (child's pose) to cultivate inner stability and conserve energy.

Join Yoga with Adriene in this alternate nostril breathing practice.
(*Scan QR code*)

2.39

Aparigrahā sthairye janmakathaṁtā saṁbodhaḥ.

Through the practice of non-possessiveness (**aparigrahā**), the yogi gains powerful perception and develops steadiness (**sthairya**).

Aparigrahā allows us to see beyond the desires of the material world. The fifth *yama*, grasping for less, and non-excess guides us to let go of the drive for over-abundance. By approaching life from a place of contentment with what is essential and a "less is more" attitude, we achieve **sthairya.** Now we perceive more clearly with *a steady gaze and a steady mind*.

The more we desire, the more we acquire. Excessiveness leads to a cluttered life filled with complicated possessions and unnecessary responsibilities. When we adopt an attitude that nothing we own truly belongs to us, we embrace the true essence of **aparigrahā.** It is with this shift that we become *human beings, not human doings*. By releasing the weight of our attachments, we find balance in our heart and peace in our soul.

By letting go of the need for accumulation and embracing a spirit of minimalism, we nurture a grounded and serene state of being. Today try shedding five things— either from your home, workplace, or mental load. With consistent practice, you will naturally stop reaching for persistent desires and shed what is not necessary. Asking yourself–do I really need this?–is a great place to begin!

Repeat the following mantra: *I release what no longer serves me. I am free from attachments, finding balance in the simplicity of being.*

Prānāyāma techniques, particularly those involving extended exhales, can aid in this process of letting go. Try it here with this practice by HeadSpace. (*Scan QR code*)

2.40 to 2.45
The 2ⁿᵈ Limb of the 8 Limb Path

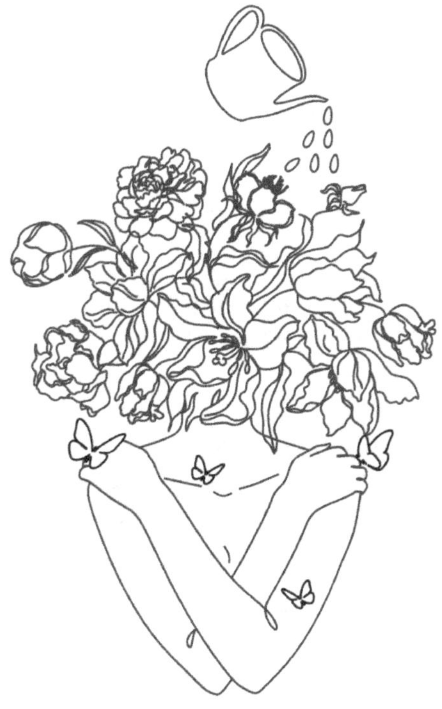

The Niyamas
Self-Care

2.40

Saucāt svāṅgajugupsā parairasaṁsargaḥ.

Through **śaucā**, self-purification and cleanliness, one learns that the body is a vessel that holds the temple of divine consciousness.

Patanjali emphasizes that our body holds the spark of the divine. It is a reminder that we should treat ourselves with reverence and care. **Saucā** is the cleanliness of every aspect of our being. The first *niyamā* can be achieved through daily hygiene practices like bathing, brushing teeth, and keeping our personal space tidy. It also involves adopting a healthy diet, mental well-being, and avoiding harmful substances.

Āyurveda, the sister science to yoga, guides us in nurturing healthy eating habits and optimizing our overall well-being by identifying our *doṣa* (dosha) type—*pitta, kapha,* or *vata.** Based on our individual personality type, it provides insights to help determine what dietary choices best serve us and lifestyle practices to align with our unique *doṣa* constitution. *Āyurveda* also offers techniques for cleansing the body and mind called shatkarmas. One such practice is using a neti pot, which cleanses the nasal passages, addressing allergies, upper respiratory issues, and other health concerns.

Other practices more traditional to India include *nauli*, a cleansing technique for massaging and strengthening the abdominal organs, and Kunjal Kriya, which involves drinking a large volume of saline water to cleanse the digestive system.

For those eager to explore the transformative self-purification practices in-depth, attending a Triguna Yoga immersion in the serene environment of Rishikesh, India, can be a life-altering journey. This immersive program presents a holistic approach to yoga, including the traditional *kriyā* self-purification techniques. (Scan QR code)

Determine your doṣa type with this questionnaire, see Appendix C: Constitution Questionnaire, page 248.

2.41

Sattva-śuddhi saumanasyaikāgryendriya-jayātma-darśana-yogyatvāni ca

Through the practice of *śaucā*, one purifies the mind. The yogi discovers peace and joy (**sattva**), one-pointedness, (**ekāgrya**), mastery over the senses (**indriya**), and insight (**darśana**) towards self-realization.

Just as dust and dirt obscure the beauty of a temple, negative thoughts and emotions clutter our minds and cloud our perception of the divinity within. **Saucā** encourages us to purify our minds from mental clutter and negativity. Through practices like *āsana*, meditation and self-awareness, we nurture the harmonious connection between body and mind.

Abhyanga, another *kriyā* for both physical and emotional benefits, is the practice of self-massage with oil. This technique supports our physical and mental relaxation while nourishing and rejuvenating the body. *Trataka*, (sūtra 1.42) also known as blinkless stare, not only cleanses and strengthens the eyes, but also improves our mental focus and concentration.

In the process of polishing within, we let go of the toxic mental patterns that impact our thoughts, words, and actions. A breath practice to clear both body and mind is *kapālabhāti* or "shining skull breath". The practice involves forcefully exhaling through the nose by drawing in the abdominal muscles followed by a natural inhale. *Kapālabhāti* is said to help improve blood circulation and oxygen levels, and to expel impurities and toxins.

When we feel healthier physically through self-purification techniques, our **sattva** glows. Try this *kriyā* practice of *kapālabhāti* with Akhanda Yoga Institute. (*Scan QR code*)

2.42

Saṁtoṣād anuttamaḥ sukha-lābhaḥ.

*From contentment, **saṁtoṣā**, unparalleled happiness (**sukha**) is attained.*

Saṁtoṣā, the second *niyama*, is the joy that blossoms when we discover that true contentment arises from the inside out, not the outside in. This internal sweetness, or **sukha**, flourishes when we are sustained and nourished by our inner abundance, rather than seeking happiness from the outside world.

Through **saṁtoṣā,** we find joy in the simple things. Our inner contentment helps us filter out harmful thought patterns, such as envy, greed, and jealousy. Instead of focusing on what we lack, we learn to appreciate what is already present with gratitude. Through our lens of abundance and love, we view the world with an optimistic outlook and seek peace in every moment.

Today, repeat the mantra:

"Nothing or nobody can bring me happiness. My happiness comes from within."

This mantra guides us when relationships or external circumstances affect us negatively. Remember that the source of true happiness does not arise from others, but from within ourselves.

For further study on discovering divine love, read *The Divine Romance* by Paramahansa Yogananda. (*Scan QR code*)

2.43

*Kāyendriya-siddhir aśuddhi-kṣayāt **tapasaḥ***

Through the practice of **tapas** (discipline), impurities of the body and the senses (**indriya**) are destroyed, leading to the attainment of great powers (**siddhis**).

Tapas, the third *niyama*, is our steady, daily commitment to cultivate restraint and burn away impurities, both physically and mentally.

Impurities include harmful emotions, habits, and attachments that hinder our spiritual progress. **Tapas** is the sacred fire and personal drive that purges these obstacles, allowing our inner strengths to flourish. This process empowers us to live a more mindful and awakened life.

To build **tapas**, commit to a disciplined *sādhana*, a daily routine of self-care rituals. From a yogic perspective discipline is not about pushing ourselves beyond our limits, but stimulating our inner strength through purification practices that serve our well-being. Daoist philosophy teaches that it takes 100 days to create a foundation—we first plant and cultivate a seed, we allow it to grow and mature for 100 days, then we reap its rewards.

Here are some practices to incorporate tapas into your life:

- Daily yoga practice and meditation.
- A day of fasting to burn excess fat and toxins.
- A day of silence without electronic devices.
- A Vipassana Meditation retreat to practice ten days of silence. (*See Additional Resources: Retreat Centers, page 292.*)
- Commit to Oprah and Deepak's 21-day meditation program. (*Scan QR code*)

2.44

Svādhyāyād iṣṭa-devatā-saṁprayogḥ.

Through study of the scriptures and self-study (**svādhyāyā**) one finds union with one's higher power.

Svādhyāyā, the fourth *niyama*, is our personal devotion to the study of spiritual texts. Through self-study, we come to better know our highest guide, our guru within, our wise intuition. Kindling our faith with this positive, supportive energy enhances our lives and our connection with the universe.

Through our yogic studies, the subtle and universal truths in and around us are revealed. Every mantra, every sound healing bowl, and every *mudrā* (hand or body gesture) invokes a certain response and serves as a guide. In recognizing that everything around us is energy, we start to witness that we are naturally drawn to certain vibrations and distance ourselves from others. If we contemplate, meditate and go inward, we will soon feel the pull and attraction to the energies that enlighten us, invoking our inner knowing of our soul's true purpose.

One such technique is the practice of a *mantra* aligned with a specific deity. *Mantras* are sacred sounds that carry the essence and energy of the deity they are associated with. The *mantra* becomes a bridge between our individual selves and the divine, creating serene inner joy with a higher power.

Chant the following *mantra* to invoke the energy of Lord Shiva, dissolving limitations and awakening the light within. (*Scan QR code*)

Om Namah Shivaya, Om Namah Shivaya, Om Namah Shivaya

I invoke the transformative power of Lord Shiva, the destroyer of ignorance, creator of wisdom, and the eternal dance of cosmic harmony.

2.45

Samādhi-siddhir īśvara-praṇidhānāt

*Through total surrender to a higher power (**īśvara praṇidhānā**) deep meditative absorption (**samādhi**) is attained.*

Iśvara praṇidhānā is the fifth *niyama*. By surrendering our ego and dedicating ourselves to our highest Self, we let go of the need for control and, in turn, embrace the present moment with openness and acceptance.

The practice of surrendering to a higher power can take many forms, depending on one's personal beliefs and values. For some, this may involve prayer or devotion to a particular deity like **Iśvara**. For others, it may involve a more abstract sense of surrender to the universe and the interconnectedness of all things.

Contemplate the wonders of the universe and ponder the following questions:

- *Where do I fit into the vastness of the cosmos?*
- *How can surrendering to a higher power help me release my attachment to outcomes and embrace the journey instead?*
- *How can I cultivate trust in the universe and let go of my need for control?*
- *How can surrendering to a higher power help me navigate challenging situations in life with grace and ease?*

Dedicate a week to reciting the mantra, *"Everything I do I offer to a higher power. My accomplishments are not my own."* Living with this truth we release our attachments and realize that everything is impermanent. We possess nothing.

2.46 to 2.48
The 3rd Limb of the 8 Limb Path

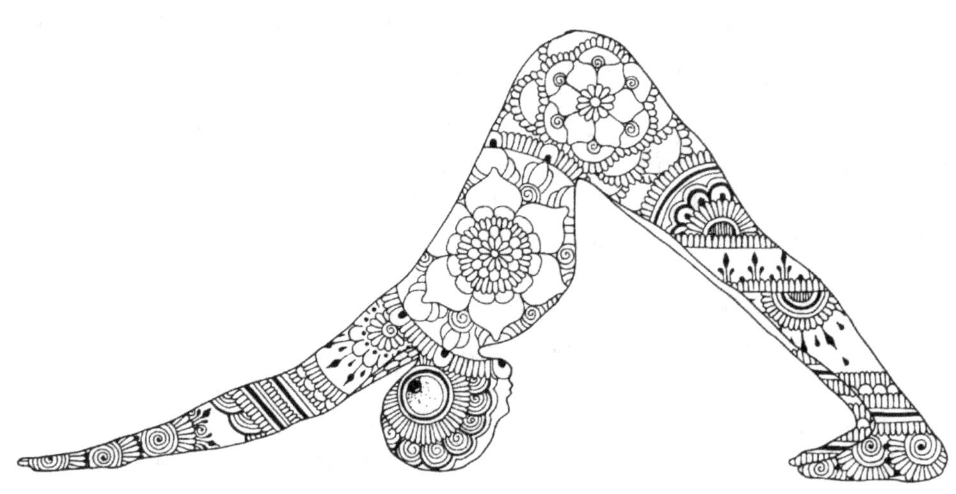

Āsana
Physical Practice

2.46
Sthira-sukham āsanam.

The physical posture (**āsana**) should be steady (**sthira**) and sweet (**sukha**).

Translating to *seat* or *posture,* **āsana** is the physical practice of yoga. Through the third limb, the yogi begins to find stillness and ease both on and off the mat.

While **āsana** practice may sometimes be regarded for its physical benefits, the ultimate goal is to nurture *sattva* through **sthira-sukham.** **Sthira** is the stability and strength found in each posture, and **sukha,** the sweetness. When **āsana** is both steady and comfortable, the yogi flows effortlessly from pose to pose, seamlessly entering a state of inner tranquility.

Āsana encompasses a wide array of postures, from still, seated positions to sweeping, dynamic movements. With many different styles of yoga available from Restorative to Ashtanga, finding a practice that leaves you feeling happy and rejuvenated is essential. Remember, an approachable and consistent practice takes precedence over intensity.

Here are some recommended classes from restorative to advanced sequencing:

Restore with Boho Beautiful
Total Body Yoga Deep Stretch, Yoga With Adriene
Advance Sequence with Dice lida-Kline. (*Scan QR code*)

2.47

Prayatna-śaithilyānanta-samāpattibhyām

Āsana is mastered by preserving one's energy and through deep meditation (**samāpatti**).

Mastery of *āsana* comes from **samāpatti,** the harmonious union of two essential elements—conservation of energy and absorption in deep meditation. Here lies the delicate balance of effort and surrender.

Yoga refines and balances the flow of *prāna* (life force energy) in the body. However, ignorance (*avidyā*) of this essential flow leads to limitations in one's practice. If *āsana* is approached with unawareness or overexertion, the yogi may never attain the gifts of the discipline. Only when we realize that the foundation of our practice lies in the quiet stillness of a moving meditation can we soar gracefully through every pose, performing even challenging postures with ease.

Throughout practice, cherish moments of returning to the breath. Return over and over again to the gentle flow of prāna as your sanctuary and focus of meditation. Each time the mind wanders gently guide your attention back. Notice the conservation of energy as your physical body softens in response. Observe how with each conscious breath you quiet the fluctuations of the mind.

With a controlled breath, a steady and comfortable body (*sthira*), and a sweet surrender (*sukha*), practice becomes what it is meant to be—a joyful moving meditation.

Practices like Tai Chi Yoga and Vinyasa flow that focus on the breath help to find this balance. Here is a Tai Chi Yoga practice with SRMD Yoga. (*Scan QR code*)

2.48
*Tato **dvandvānabhighātaḥ***

*Through the practice of the postures (āsanas) comes freedom from dualities or opposites (**dvandvā**).*

With continued practice, our actions become less determined by the influence of dualities, such as good or bad, pleasure and pain, thin or fat, or happiness and sadness. By engaging in *āsana*, we transcend the black and white, oppositional thinking known as **dvandvā,** and start to recognize the infinite shades of life awakening within us.

Consider those moments on your yoga mat when you judged yourself as "good" or "bad". In the past, you may have evaluated yourself by your performance in each pose, labeling yourself as good when executing a pose perfectly and bad when you struggled or fell short of expectations. Our self-judgment creates a sense of division and limitation in our *sadhana,* but as our practice expands, so does our perspective. Through *āsana*, rather than being preoccupied with external standards and flawless appearances, we stay true to our path, resilient in the face of critiques and comparisons, and experience the transformative power of showing up.

As we shift internally, each pose becomes an opportunity for self-exploration and self-acceptance. We start to experience that yoga is not about achieving perfection or conforming to external standards. Rather, it is a practice of connecting with our body, breath, and inner self. Through experience, we free ourselves from the constraints of judgment and dualistic thinking and embrace an expansive perspective that extends beyond the mat and into everyday life.

Explore a non-dualistic approach with *Nondual Guided Meditation* by Shamash. (*Scan QR code*)

2.49 to 2.53
The 4th Limb of the 8 Limb Path

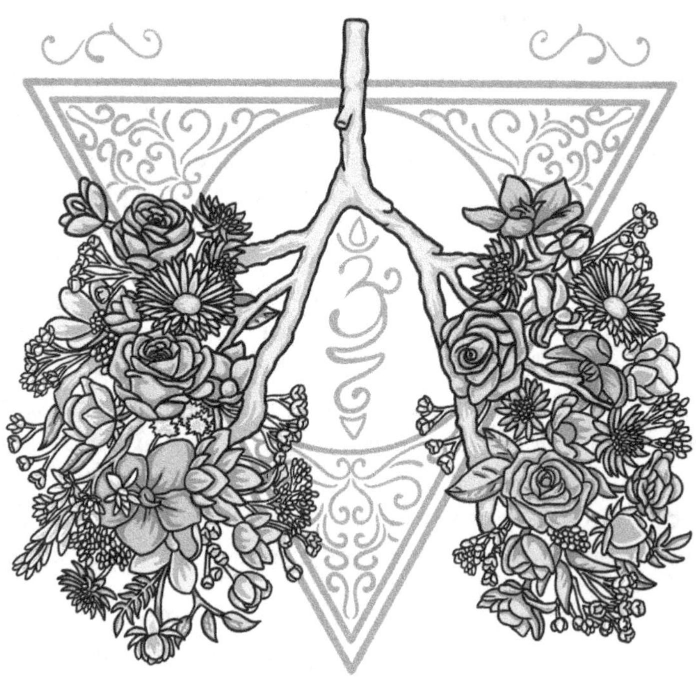

Prāṇāyāma
Breathing Techniques

2.49

*Tasmin sati śvāsa-praśvāsayor gati-vichchhedaḥ **prāṇāyāmaḥ***

Prāṇāyāma is the control of the inhalation and exhalation of breath.

For thousands of years, yogis have understood that mastery of the breath leads to mastery of the mind. This was noted in the *Bhagavad Gita,* and later in the 15th-century text, the *Hatha Yoga Pradipika,* which teaches that when the ***prāṇa*** is still, the mind is still. From Sanskrit, ***prāṇa*** translates to "life force" or "vital energy," and ***yāma*** to "restraint" or "control". ***Prāṇāyāma***, the fourth limb, is the conscious and intentional regulation of breath to enhance the flow of ***prāṇa*** in the body.

Modern science confirms the validity of these ancient beliefs. ***Prāṇāyāma*** significantly impacts our physiology and overall health. Breathwork reduces stress and anxiety, lessens pain, and awakens the parasympathetic nervous system. In addition, the science of positive psychology is leveraging breathwork to help people connect to their strengths of character in order to live more engaged and fulfilling lives thereby improving their mental health.

Consider the lifespan of a turtle, which can exceed 200 years. This longevity is attributed to their slower rate of respiration. While we may never attain such a lengthy lifespan, we can deepen our breath and our practice through the exploration of different ***prāṇāyāma*** techniques like *ujjayi* (oceanic or victory breath), *kapālabhāti* (shining skull breath), or *nāḍī shodhana* (alternate nostril breathing).

To start, engage in this *3-Minute Breathwork Practice* with positive psychology author Fatima Doman to connect with your authentic self, illuminating your strengths of character to boost life satisfaction and fulfillment. (*Scan QR code*)

2.50

*Bāhyābhyantara-stambha-vṛttiḥ **deśakāla-saṅkhyābhiḥ** paridṛṣṭo dirgha-**sūkṣmaḥ***

Prāṇāyāma is the regulation of the inhale and exhale. By bringing focus to the location (**deśa**), time (**kāla**), and count (**saṅkhyā**) of the breath, our **prāna** expands and becomes more subtle (**sūkṣma**).

Here are three examples of **prāṇāyāma** practices based on place, time and length of breath:

Deśa (place of focus): *Bring your awareness to the tip of your nose. Observe the sensation of air flowing in and out of your nostrils. Hold your attention here for a few moments, then shift your awareness to the rise and fall of your chest. Notice the changing sensations here, then move to observe the flow of **prāna** from the abdomen. Continue this practice and watch how quickly the mind calms.*

Kāla (amount of time): Breathing in and out through the nose, *inhale for one count followed by an exhale for one count. Continuing to breathe in and out through the nose, next, inhale for one count and exhale for two counts. Then, inhale for one count and exhale for three counts. Continue the sequence up to eight counts of exhalation.*

Saṅkhyā (Length or count): *Explore different breathing ratios, such as inhaling for four counts and exhaling for six, or inhaling for six counts and exhaling for eight.*

Learn more by exploring the contemporary books *Breath* by James Nestor, *The Science of Breath* by Swami Rama, *The Yoga of Breath* by Richard Rosen, *The Breathing Book* by Donna Farhi, or *Body by Breath* by Jill Miller. (*Scan QR code*)

2.51

Bāhyābhyantaraviṣayākṣepi chaturthaḥ

A fourth *prānāyāma* practice transcends the internal and external realms.

Through *āsana* practice, we become free from *dvandvā* (*sūtra* 2.48) or dualities. This includes the perception of separation between the inner and outer realms. Now, the inhale flows seamlessly into the exhale, and the exhale seamlessly into the inhale.

The breath cycle consists of four parts: *puraka* (the inhale), *rechaka* (the exhale), and the suspension of breath (*kumbhaka*) that immediately follows the inhalation and the exhalation. By exploring the practice of an uninterrupted cycle of breath in this fourth *prānāyāma*, we discover there is no real distinction between parts. The boundless, continuous flow of *prānā* moves beyond labels and awakens realms of being that transcend the internal and the external. Often practiced in Kundalini yoga, the fourth *prānāyāma* utilizes powerful techniques to awaken higher consciousness.

Come to your seat, lengthen your spine and bring your hands to your knees. Take an inhale through the nose as you lift the chest towards the sky. Exhale through the mouth with pursed lips and a strong audible sound. As you exhale round the back. Repeat this pattern continuing to coordinate your intense breath with the movement of your body. Sense the inhale and exhale as one continuous flow of prānā.

Try this advanced practice called *Awakening Cosmic Consciousness* (Cosmic Breath) with Sattva Connect. (*Scan QR code*)

2.52

*Tataḥ kṣiyate **prakāśā**varaṇam*

Through *prānāyāma,* the dark veil over the illuminated self (***prakāśā***) is lifted allowing the inner light of awareness to shine.

To transform *maya* (the illusion of the material world) and attune ourselves with the brilliance of consciousness (***prakāśā***), we must remove the barriers that obscure the union of *puruṣa* and *prakṛti,* of the spirit and the material. Through the diligent practice of *prānāyāma,* we begin to dissolve this veil and allow the innate brilliance of our true nature to shine forth.

Breathwork is instrumental in breaking free from the grip of the *klesās* and the on-going cycle of *karma.* As we harness the power of breath control, we experience a shift in our being that frees us from the entanglements of *samsāra*–the journey of the spirit through birth, death, and rebirth.

Wim Hof is an inspiring example of the transformative power of *prānāyāma.* Through his intense breathing techniques, he has achieved remarkable feats, such as staying submerged in ice water for over 20 minutes. His methods have also been shown to help people with various health challenges, including autoimmune disorders, arthritis, and depression[1].

If you want to take your pranayama practice to the next level, try this advanced breathing practice. (*Scan QR code*)

2.53

Dhāraṇā su cha yogyata manasa

*Prāṇāyāma readies one for concentration—**dhāraṇā** (the 6th limb of yoga).*

With the steady practice of *prāṇāyāma* prolonged periods of focus and concentration known as **dhāraṇā** begin to emerge. This centered state fosters the ability to retain **prāṇā** for extended lengths of time. The rishis teach that the breath may stop for several minutes without causing harm to the body, for in this state of deep concentration, **prāṇā** is being preserved, rather than wasted.

Milarepa, a Tibetan Buddhist, was renowned for his extraordinary breath control. During his years of intense meditation and solitary retreats in the mountains, he would enter states of deep absorption where his breath would naturally cease. He would remain in this breathless state for extended periods, sustaining his life force through inner energy and spiritual nourishment[2].

While achieving such extraordinary states may be rare, the regular practice of *prāṇāyāma* brings increased focus, clarity, and a deeper connection to our vital life energy.

*Close your eyes and bring your awareness to your breath. Keep the focus here and take a full-body inhale followed by a full-body exhale. At the bottom of the exhale hold the breath without tension. As you hold the breath imagine, prāṇā flowing through every cell of your body. Breathing deeply and consciously take another full-body inhale and full-body exhale and continue this pattern. Remember as you hold the breath to feel the flow of prāṇā coursing through your entire being. Notice the **dhāraṇā** emerging.*

Explore the transformative power of *prāṇāyāma* by SRMD Yoga. (*Scan QR code*)

2.54 to 2.55
The 5ᵗʰ Limb of the 8 Limb Path

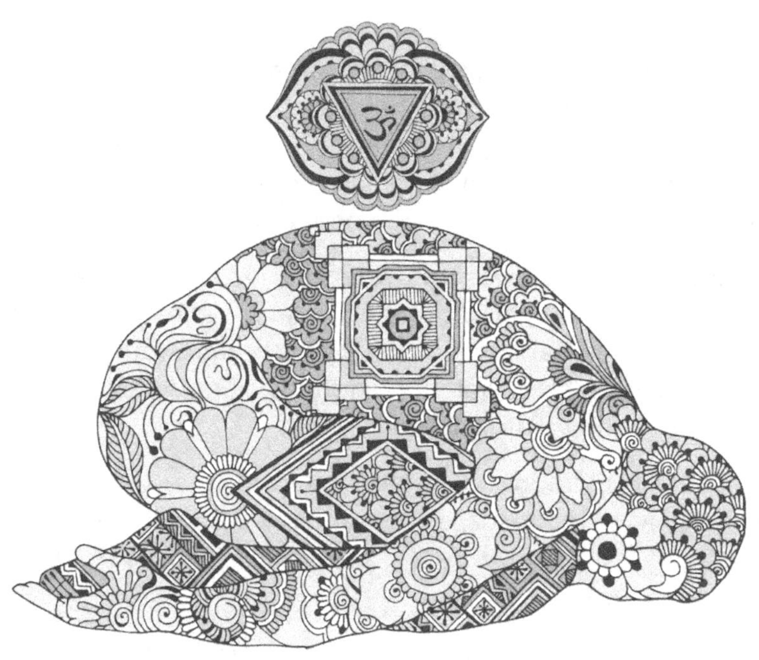

Pratyāhāra
Withdrawing the Senses

2.54

*Svaviṣayāsaṃprayoge **citta**syasvarūpānukāra ivendriyāṇām **pratyāhāraḥ***

Pratyāhāra is the withdrawal of the senses from external objects. As the mind draws inward, the senses assume the form of their own true Nature.

2.55

*tataḥ paramā vaśyate**ndriyāṇām***

By practicing, we gain control over our senses (**indriyas**).

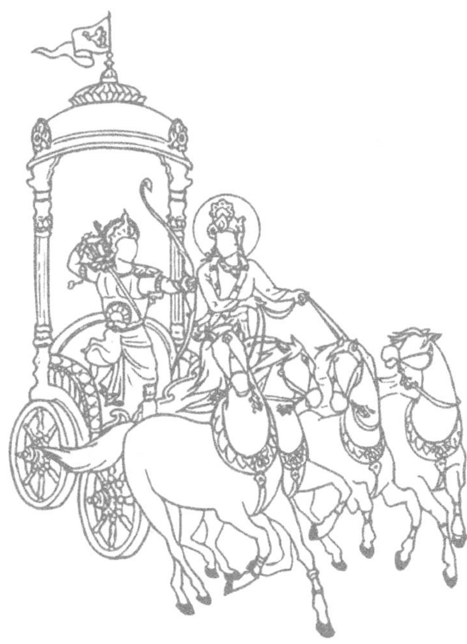

Pratyāhāra, the fifth limb, is the conscious letting go of sensory stimuli. This practice frees us from the constant external distractions through sight, sound, touch, taste, and smell. Through **pratyāhāra** we develop mastery over our mind and become more focused and less distracted, which in turn moves us further along the path.

The classic epic poem the *Bhagavad Gita** illustrates the essence of **pratyāhāra.** The hero, Arjuna, rides into a fierce battle with his passenger and guide Krishna, supreme consciousness personified. Together they guide their chariot fearlessly, but with uncertainty, along the front line. In this allegory, Arjuna symbolizes the Self and his five chariot horses represent the five senses.

Through his dialogue with Krishna, Arjuna turns inward and discovers great wisdom. He comes to understand that the divine alone is the guide, the one who drives his chariot and his *karma*. Like Arjuna and his horses, as we gain wisdom, we recognize our ability to restrain our senses, and direct our mind and focus towards higher pursuits.

Bhramari prānāyāma, humming bee breath, is a practice for developing **pratyāhāra.** *"Cover" your senses by putting your thumbs gently over your ears, your index fingers and middle fingers over the eyes, the ring fingers along the nostrils and little fingers gently over the lips. While doing so, make a humming sound. Notice how your mind calms as your focus is redirected inward, reducing attachment to external sensory distractions. (Scan QR code)*

** The Bhagavad Gita is one section of the full work, The Mahabharata, considered the longest epic poem ever written—it is nearly three times the length of the bible. It recounts the story of two royal families, the Pandavas and the Kauravas and their ongoing conflicts.*

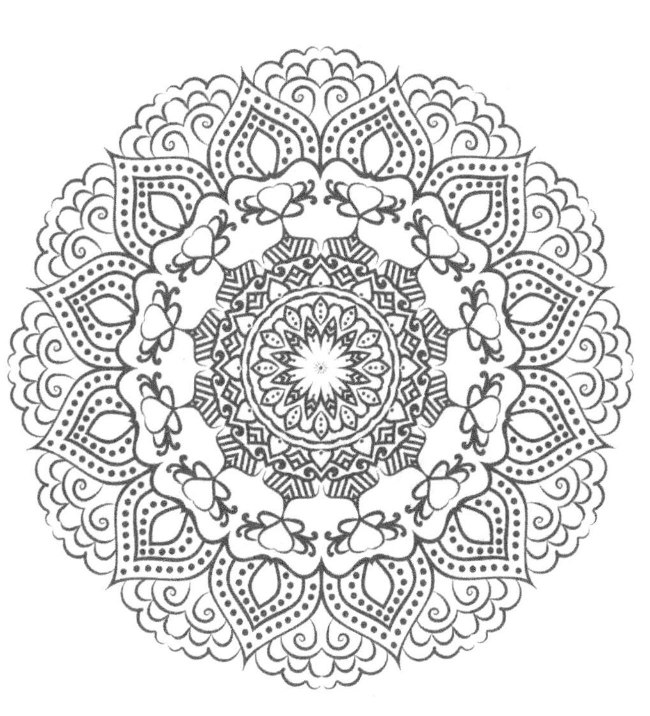

Chapter Three
Vibhūti Pāda
The Path to Extraordinary Powers

Pāda Three explores the extraordinary gifts of yoga, known as **vibhūtis** or *siddhis*. These mystic abilities may appear at first like inconceivable superpowers, but remain open with curiosity to discover all that is achievable through dedicated practice. Just like the infinite possibilities in the mysteries of our vast universe, from its countless galaxies to the miraculous diversity of life on our tiny Earth, these *siddhis* invite us to delve deeper into the equally infinite dimensions of the human mind.

- The Advanced Limbs of Yoga: Dhāraṇā-Dhyāna-Samādhi (3.1 to 3.3)
- Saṁyama: Union of the Final 3 Limbs (3.4 to 3.8)
- Pariṇāma: Transformation (3.9 to 3.15)
- Vibhūti or Siddhis (3.16 to 3.49)
  - 3.16 to 3.26 – Siddhis of Jñāna, Sattva, and Manas: Mastery of Wisdom, Spirit, and Mind
  - 3.27 to 3.29 – Siddhis: On the Miracles of the Universe
  - 3.30 to 3.39 – Siddhis of the Inner Channels
  - 3.40 to 3.45 – Siddhis of the Vayus: Mastery of the Inner Winds
  - 3.46 – The Eight Mystical Siddhis
  - 3.47 to 3.49 – The Qualities of the Siddha: Attaining Perfection and Freedom
- 3.50 to 3:52 – The End of Wordly Attachment
- 3.53 to 3.56 – Viveka Jñāna: Divine Knowledge

3.1 to 3.3
The Advanced Limbs of Yoga
Dhāraṇā-Dhyāna-Samādhi

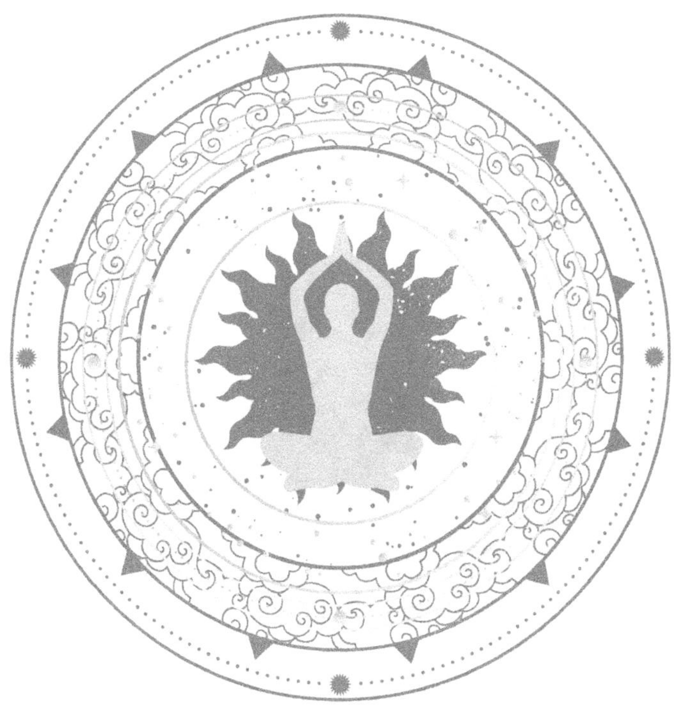

I have been a seeker and I still am, but I stopped asking the books
and the stars. I started listening to the teaching of my Soul.

- Rumi -

3.1
The 6ᵗʰ Limb of the 8 Limb Path

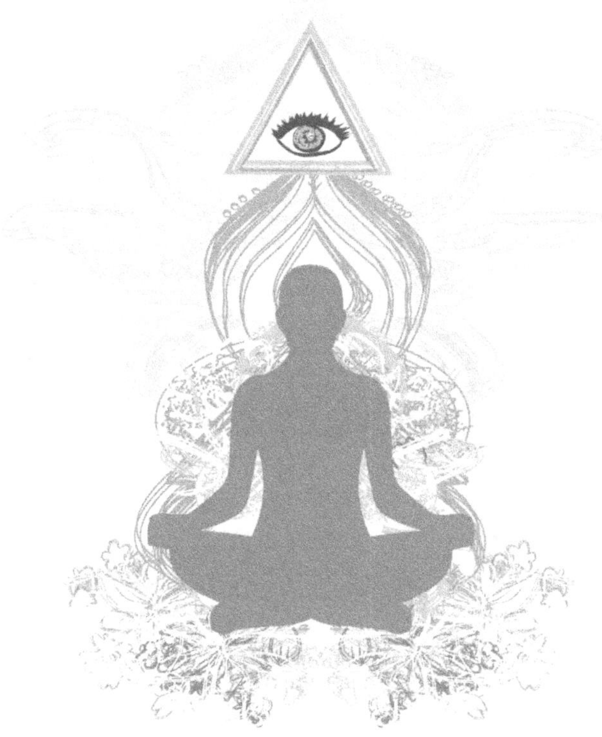

Dhāraṇā
Concentration

3.1
Deśa-bandhaś cittasya dhāraṇā

Dhāraṇā is the practice of binding the mind to one place (**deśa-bandha**).

Dhāraṇā, the sixth limb, is the practice of concentration. The action of **dhāraṇā** involves holding the mind unwaveringly on a chosen point, idea or activity. This focal point is a **deśa-bandha**, or more commonly referred to as a *dristi*. Through the discipline found in practicing concentration, the mind becomes grounded, less likely to be swayed by distractions, and more adept at accessing deep levels of absorption.

Dhāraṇā, though is a journey. It is normal for the mind to wander, and to be swayed by *vikṣepa*, the oscillating rhythm of mental fluctuations. When these distractions arise, grant yourself grace and gently guide your attention back to your *dṛṣṭi*.

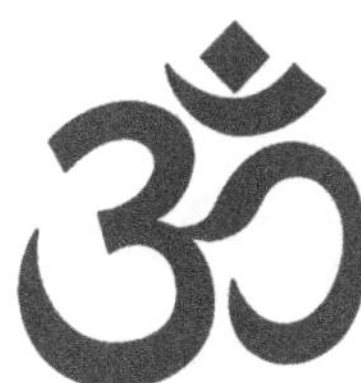

Over time, the mind learns to hold steadfast to its anchor point.

Come to a meditative seat and concentrate on the OM symbol above. Observe its soft lines and contours. Close your eyes and see the symbol's silhouette in your mind's eye. Hold this vision as your inner dṛṣṭi. When the form fades from view, gently open your eyes and gaze again at the symbol. Envision OM, and allow your eyes to close once more. Notice how time fades, and how, with practice, its divine essence expands your concentration.

3.2
The 7ᵗʰ Limb of the 8 Limb Path

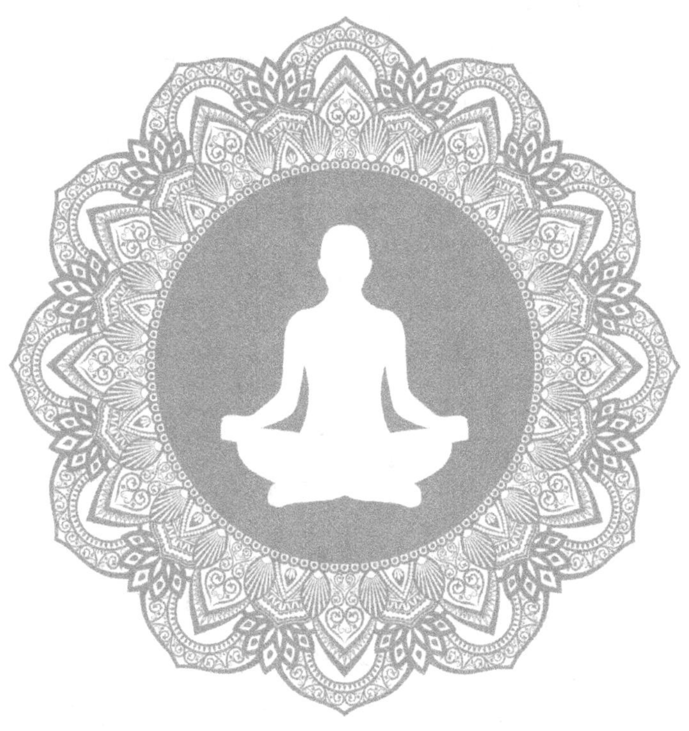

Dhyāna
Meditation

3.2
*Tatra pratyayaika-tānatā **dhyānam***

Meditation (**dhyāna**) is the uninterrupted flow of one-pointed attention towards a single focus.

We have all experienced moments when we were so fully immersed in an activity, minutes or even hours passed unnoticed. In **dhyāna**, the seventh limb, meditation, the mind is so clear, peaceful and focused in the flow of moments that time slips away. The practice of *dhāraṇā*, concentration, now natural flows into **dhyāna**, uninterrupted absorption in an object or activity of focus.

Whether our meditation takes the form of a still seat, the repetition of a mantra, the continuous flow of *asāna*, or even an activity such as dance, when we enter into a state of *sattva* filled with peace and dissolution of time, this is **dhyāna**.

To encourage your personal meditation, find a space in your home that inspires tranquility. Fill the space with sacred objects, comfortable bolsters, or an altar of devotion. Maybe choose to include pictures of your personal gurus or loved ones. This space will serve as a daily physical reminder that inspires you to find your comfortable seat.

Here is one form of meditation using the mantra "I Love You":

Close your eyes and take a few deep breaths. Each time a thought arises, say internally, "I love you." No matter the incoming feeling, offer it love. As different people or events enter your mind, say "I love you", even to those you find challenging. Let the hum of "I love you" welcome all and become your uplifting mantra. With practice, try carrying this meditation with you as you move about your day, enjoying its calming effect.

Continue the practice with this meditation. (*Scan QR code*)

3.3
The 8ᵗʰ Limb of the 8 Limb Path

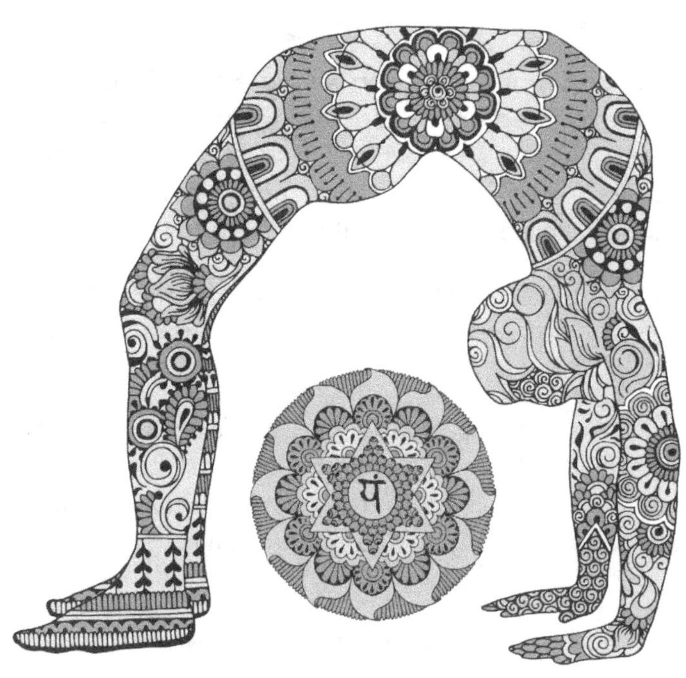

Samādhi
Absorption

3.3

*Tad evārtha-mātra-nirbhāsam **svarūpa-śūnyam** iva **samādhiḥ***

In samādhi, the essence of the object shines alone in the *citta*, and the mind empties itself (**śūnya**) of its own self-awareness.

The eighth and final limb, **samādhi,** meditative absorption brings us to the ultimate practice on the path. When every moment of our day, including life's ordinary tasks, reflects a continuous state of meditation (*dhyāna*), this is where **samādhi** begins.

With the fluctuating waves of the *citta* at rest, the richness of life unfolds. Rather than exerting control in our pursuits, each moment now flows effortlessly into a state of non-doing. We let the universe move through us remaining absorbed in the Now. The boundaries between the meditator and the process of meditation begin to blur, and the mind, now emptied (**śūnya**), radiates with the brilliance of cosmic consciousness–**samādhi**.

*Take a few deep breaths to settle. Close your eyes and begin to chant OM. Bring your awareness to the resonance of the sound. With each repetition, allow the boundaries between each arising vibration to dissolve. Continue to chant until you have merged with the pulsation of OM. When all that remains is the brilliance of the sound, notice how the awareness of your own existence gets carried away by the flow of the present moment. Sense the emptiness of the mind, or **śūnya**, making space for eternal Joy, where the boundaries between the self and object dissolve entirely.*

Enhance your meditation with this OM playlist. Allow the sound to guide you into a state of complete absorption. (*Scan QR code*)

3.4 to 3.8
Saṁyama
The Union of Dhāranā, Dhyāna, and Samādhi

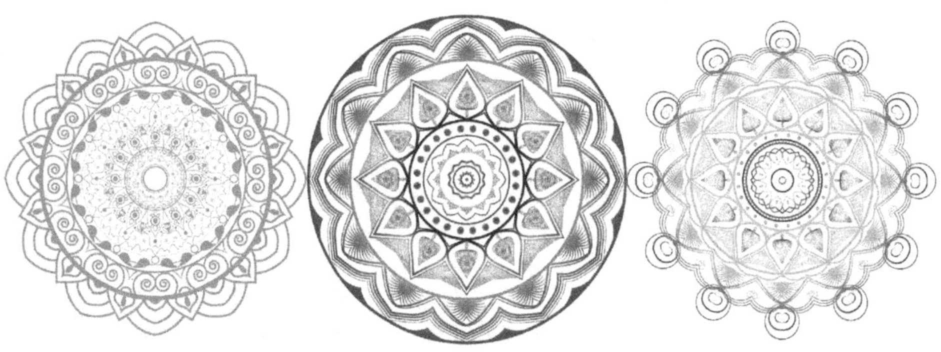

You do not need to seek freedom in some distant land for everything already exists within your own body, heart, mind and soul.

- B.K.S. Iyengar -

3.4
Trayam ekatra saṁyamḥ

Saṁyama is the unified application of the final three limbs (*dhāraṇā, dhyāna,* and *samādhi*) on one-pointedness (**ekatra**).

By combining concentration, meditation and absorption, the possibility of reaching higher states of consciousness begins to unfold. Through this integrated practice innate wisdom, creativity, and intuition flourish. It is here where the possibility of *siddhis* begins.

Think of **saṁyama** like the process a scientist uses to uncover the facts of sub-atomic structures. Only with intense study, focus, and complete absorption can they decode the intricacies hidden within the subtlest aspects of existence. As a scientist unravels the secrets of the universe through increasingly refined methods of experimentation, the yogi, through the practice of **saṁyama** peers into the deepest recesses of consciousness and reality.

As though you were conducting an experiment of self-discovery, explore the terrain of your being. Observe your body, releasing any feelings of tension. Observe your breath as your dṛṣṭi, and notice if it is peaceful or restricted. Observe your mind and the thoughts that come and go without judgment.

Keep steady focus on the mind and envision the full moon in your skull. Hold to this internal vision until it shines in the citta. Notice how the lines between the observer and what is being observed begin to blur. Embody this harmonious union of the present moment.

Practice unwavering focus with *Yin Yoga To Go Inward & Retreat* by The Bare Female and *Yoga for Deep Focus,* Patrick Beach. (*Scan QR code*)

3.5
*Tajjayāt **prajñālokḥ***

By practicing *samyama*, deep wisdom (**prajñā**) is illuminated (**ālok**).

Through *samyama*, our inner light–*alokḥ*–is awakened. Different from *jyoti*, (sūtra 1.36), this brilliance transcends the limitations of the mind. It emanates from deep within the subtlest layers of our being that lie beyond intellectual understanding. With the awakening of **ālokḥ**, the mind stills, illuminating higher realms of comprehension to guide us towards the boundless wisdom of the universe.

Enlightened by **prajñālokḥ**, it is easy to see beyond the veils of illusion or *maya* and perceive the true nature of things. With clear discernment, we make thoughtful decisions, nurture intuition, and attune to the subtle energies and deeper truths beneath the surface of our experiences. Now, ignorance and confusion are replaced with divine knowledge and enhanced clarity.

*Find a mindful seat and gently close your eyes. Softly gaze into your Third Eye space between the eyebrows and connect with the luminous glow radiating from within. As you take a full body inhale, allow the light to emanate from your heart and rise to the seat of wisdom at your Third Eye. Continue as you sense this luminous light, inhaling from the heart to the Third Eye, and exhaling from the Third Eye back to the heart. Feel the expansive flow of light, harmonizing with each breath. Continue this rhythmic sequence, allowing the mind to quiet with each cycle. As the luminous glow envelops you, open yourself to the **prajñālokḥ** that arises.*

Continue this practice with *Inner Light Breathing- Meditation* by Cory Cochiolo, Insight Timer. (*Scan QR code*)

3.6
*Tasya **bhūmiṣu** viniyogḥ*

The practice (**viniyogh**) of *saṁyama* is applied in stages (**bhūmi**)

In the initial stages, a yogi may focus on mastering the physical aspects of practice, dedicating time to perfecting the postures, movement and breath. Through *abhyā-sa* (discipline) and *vairāgya* (letting go), we are drawn to deeper levels of practice as we witness the ever-changing nature of our being. As our minds settle we move forward with the advanced practices. In the next half of our journey, attention advances to aligning the mind and body with divine spirit, moving from the tangible to the ethereal.

Ascending the rungs of the ladder of consciousness, we advance in **bhūmi** *or* stages. When new heights of progress are reached, new insights are revealed that gradually unravel the many subtle layers of awareness that govern the mind. This practice nurtures and enriches the ever-expanding journey towards self-realization.

Become the architect of your own metamorphosis and embrace each rung with faith, patience and perseverance. Revisit past teachings and stay open to the new dimensions of awareness they now reveal. Let the union of concentration, meditation and *samādhi* fill your spirit as the practice gradually unfolds the beautiful essence of your divine Self.

Step into the depths of your being with this Mooji meditation, *You Are Silence Itself*. (*Scan QR code*).

3.7

Trayam antaraṅgam pūrvebhyḥ.

The final three limbs are more internal and subtle than the previous.

The eight limbs form a hierarchical progression guiding the yogi from the external to internal realms. The depth of consciousness unfolding goes even deeper with the final three limbs—*dhāraṇā, dhyāna,* and *samādhi.*

Try a comprehensive practice incorporating all eight limbs of yoga. Begin with the yamas (ethical principles) and observe your interactions with others and the world. Reflect on the 5 yamas of non-harming, truthfulness, non-stealing, conservation of energy and non-clinging. Move to the niyamas (observances) and examine your self-care practices and study of the yogic texts. Do you feed your body with food that enhances your wellbeing? What are you reading and watching? Does it contribute to your personal growth?

Transition to the third limb, āsana, by flowing through sun salutations, establishing a connection between breath and movement. Proceed to prāṇāyāma, and explore breath control techniques such as lengthening the exhale. Then, practice pratyāhāra by sitting quietly and gently withdrawing your senses from external distractions.

Engage in dhāraṇā, the sixth limb, by focusing your attention on a chosen object or mantra, allowing your mind to find single-pointedness. Moving into the seventh limb, dhyāna, experience a sense of timelessness and spacelessness, where the subject and object merge in meditation. Conclude the practice with the recitation of "OM", submerging yourself in its internal resonance and sealing the journey with a sense of sacred unity—samādhi.

3.8
*Tad api bahir-aṅgam **nirbīja**sya*

Even these final limbs are external compared to [internal] **nirbīja samādhi** (that which is without seed or object).

The unified practice of concentration, meditation and **samādhi** nurtures a serene inner peace, yet the mind may still grow bored and wander. This union of the final three limbs is a state of *samprajñata samādhi* (1.17) where an external point of focus or seed remains. There are still more states of meditation to discover beyond this union.

In the deeper *asamprajñata samādhi*, meditation is **nirbīja**, or without seed. *In **nirbīja samādhi*** the mind is empty (**śūnya**) and rests in its own true nature. Now the *citta* is completely free. Rooted in its own soil, the Self blossoms, undisturbed by the fluctuations of the mind. Our journey is now unburdened from the anxieties of the future or the heaviness of past regrets.

In this stage of absorption, guidance flows freely from the reservoir of wisdom beyond the rational mind (3.5), and peace is our constant companion through our daily challenges. Now we recognize the impermanence of worldly pursuits and escape from our need for external validation.

With **nirbīja** we gain resilience in adversity and, most importantly, clarity towards our *dharma*, our life's purpose.

Explore the state of **nirbīja samādhi** with *Pure Awareness I Am* by Mooji.
(*Scan QR code*)

3.9 to 3.15
Parināma
Transformation

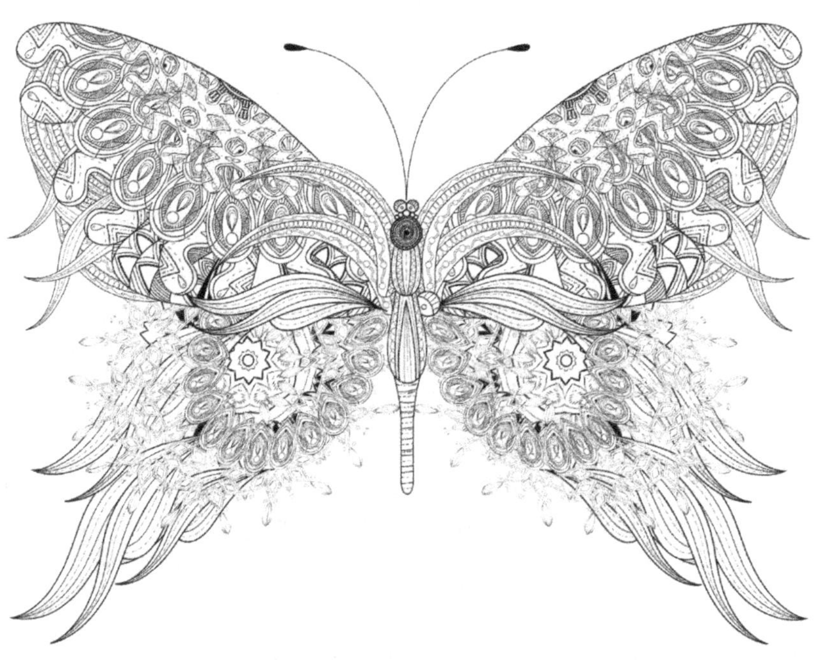

Change Yourself and you have done your part
in changing the world.
- *Paramahansa Yogananda* -

3.9

*Vyutthāna-**nirodha-saṁskāra**yor-abhibhava-prādurbhāvau*
*nirodha-kṣaṇa-cittānvayo **nirodha-pariṇāmaḥ***

Nirodha-Pariṇāma is the transformation that takes place when emerging mental impressions (**saṁskāras**) dissolve rather than stir the mind.

3.10

*Tasya praśānta vāhitā **saṁskārā**t*

When the mind is in a state of a peaceful flow, it is because the **saṁskārās** are quieted and subdued.

3.11

*Sarvārthatai**kāgratayoḥ** kṣayodayau **cittasya samādhi-pariṇāmḥ***

Consequently, after the wandering mind is destroyed, one-pointedness (**ekāgratā**) follows. This transformation of the mind is **samādhi-pariṇāma**.

Through deeper states of meditation (**nirodha-pariṇāma**), we release the mental fluctuations (*vṛittis*) and ingrained patterns (**saṁskārās**) that obstruct our spiritual growth. Cultivating clarity and purity of mind through *saṁyama* helps us build an internal warehouse of positive impressions. Through transformation (**pariṇāma**), once disruptive **saṁskārās** are now tranquil and subdued.

In yoga we chant *Om shanti, shanti, shanti, Om* meaning "I am eternal peace, peace, peace." When true peace is attained, when it is experienced over and over again through meditation, then **ekāgratā pariṇāma** arises and the yogi remains undisturbed even in the face of adversity.

Our brains possess a remarkable ability to evolve, contradicting any notion of being doomed or permanently stuck. According to Swami Satyananda Saraswati in *Four Chapters on Freedom*, in these advanced stages of meditation the molecular structure of the mind changes. Modern science confirms this phenomenon, calling it neuroplasticity.

Meditation and other mindful practices offer hope and empowerment to those seeking positive change in their lives. Through mindful practices our brains undergo structural metamorphosis and just like the caterpillar who transforms into a butterfly, we too can transform our being.

Watch as a caterpillar turns itself into a butterfly. Reflect on this miracle of nature as you self-unfold through yoga. (*Scan QR code*)

3.12

*tataḥ punaḥ śāntoditau tulya**pratyay**au citta**syaikāgratā pariṇāmaḥ***

One-pointed (**ekāgratā**) transformation is when subsiding and arising perceptions are identical from one moment to the next.

Like a cosmic dance, subsiding and arising, with **ekāgratā pariṇāma** perceptions become one seamless wave, effortlessly flowing in perfect rhythm. Now, the constraints of past and future thoughts dissolve, and distractions that typically cloud the mind are dispelled.

Time and space disappear as the void between thoughts expands into an ocean of stillness. With **ekāgratā**, we become attuned to the cosmic dance of existence, and move in sync with its universal flow.

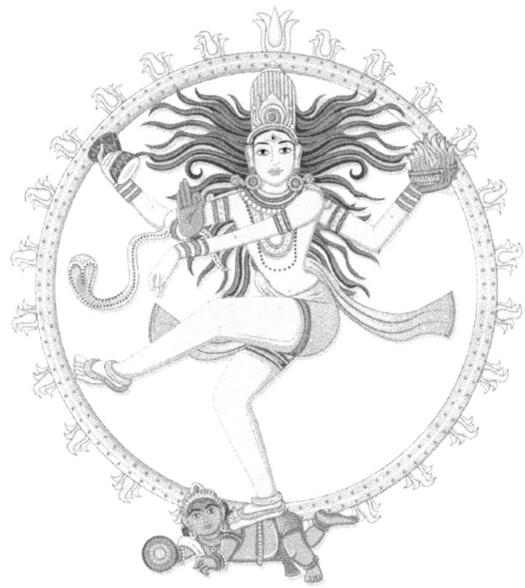

Shiva Nataraja is the cosmic dancer, representing divine consciousness and Bliss. His dance embodies the rhythm of the universe and the eternal cycle of creation, preservation, and dissolution. Standing upon a human figure in his statue form, Shiva stamps out all impurities, obstacles and *saṁskāras*. Shiva reminds us to step into the flow of the universe and become attuned to the rhythm of our being.

The next time you come to your mat, imagine Shiva dancing in the cosmos and feel the resonance of his eternal rhythm. Allow any distractions to dissolve, recognizing them as mere ripples in the vast ocean of your inner peace. Sense the effortless flow of Shiva's dance, a cosmic ballet that mirrors the continuous cycle of birth, life, death and rebirth. With each graceful step, feel your connection to universal energy, embracing the unwavering stillness within the eternal dance of existence.

Repeat the mantra:

I flow with the rhythm of life. I flow with the rhythm of life. Whatever comes my way, I flow with the rhythm of life.

Explore Shiva dancing in the cosmos with this Shiva inspired class by Megan at Yogatrotter. (*Scan QR code*)

3.13

Etena **bhūtendriyeṣu dharma lakṣaṇāvasthā pariṇāmā** *vyākhyātāḥ.*

Consequently, there is transformation of characteristics, state and condition of the elements including one's own being.

At this stage of *pariṇāmā*, it's easy to see that everything is in flux, including our bodies and our senses (**indriyas**). While the practice of *saṁyama* initiates change, there are of course inevitable transformations beyond our control.

Numerous factors contribute to the transformations we experience in our lives, however, Patanjali chooses to draw our attention to three specific types of *pariṇāma*:

1. *Dharma pariṇāma* – when the defining characteristics of a being transform in their fundamental nature, like a caterpillar transforming into a butterfly.

2. *Lakṣaṇā pariṇāma* – when there are state changes or perceivable effects caused by time or environment, such as getting older with age.

3. *Avasthā pariṇāma* – when the change in nature or being comes to full maturity, such as a fruit reaching its peak ripeness and then decaying.

Through *saṁyama*, we learn that everything we do impacts how our biological processes develop. Our purpose, environment, and our maturity impact the choices we make and affect our progress towards spiritual growth.

By concentrating on our daily practice of meditation, our *saṁyama* holds the capacity to influence our evolution and the cycle of growth, decay and rebirth. While certain changes remain outside of our control, by making an effort towards living in a *sattvic* way, yoga builds habits that support our constant evolution towards Freedom.

3.14

*Śāntoditāvyapadeśya **dharmānupātī dharmī.***

While all these transformations take place, the underlying net of the true self (**dharmī**) remains constant throughout Time.

While everything within us and around us is evolving or has the potential to evolve, something remains constant. This is the substratum, the **dharmī.**

Imagine **dharmī** as the canvas on which a painter creates a work of art. The colors and shapes may transform with each stroke of the brush, yet the canvas itself remains a constant foundation for the ever-changing work of art. Similarly, while experiences, emotions, and events reflect a diverse tapestry of life, **dharmī** is the unwavering canvas behind our ever-changing existence.

As we face various challenges and experiences, solace can always be found by returning to our seat on the mat to realign with our **dharmī.** Our inner space becomes our sanctuary to sit with what is changeless. Here, we peel away the layers of our being, along with the conditioning and fears that may have obscured our true purpose, and settle into the steady, unchanging aspect of ourselves.

For those shrouded in the constant flux of *citta-vṛtti*-ing, discovering our **dharma** can be an ongoing struggle. However, after we grant ourselves the freedom to unfold our true Nature, our personal magic radiates from the substratum. Aglow, our **dharma** becomes the driving force that infuses our life with meaning and direction, allowing us to skillfully embrace a path that resonates with our authentic Self.

3.15

Kramānyatvam pariṇāmānyatve hetuḥ.

Successive sequence (**kramā**) is the cause of transformation (**pariṇāmā**).

Just like a seed that gradually grows into a majestic tree, our evolution requires patience and nurturing. Patanjali reminds us that a steady, consistent practice over time allows for a deeper and more sustainable transformation. For example, a committed practice of 20 minutes a day may be more effective in manifesting long-term change than attending a weeklong "transformative" retreat.

Repetition shapes our external behavior and also rewires our internal patterns creating new neural pathways. More simply said, by repeating a positive action, again and again, healthy habits become ingrained in our being.

Identify a behavior or habit that you would like to transform. Break it down into small steps or stages and create a plan to gradually progress. If you want to develop a daily meditation practice, try starting with just a few minutes a day.

Gradually increase the time over several weeks or months, and it will become a natural part of your daily routine. Even Olympic athletes are not born overnight. It takes steady, unwavering burning desire and practice (tapas and abhyāsa). Small consistent effort will lead to lasting transformation.

Be inspired with Caro Arevalos' daily commitment to yoga. (*Scan QR code*)

3.16 to 3.49
Siddhis

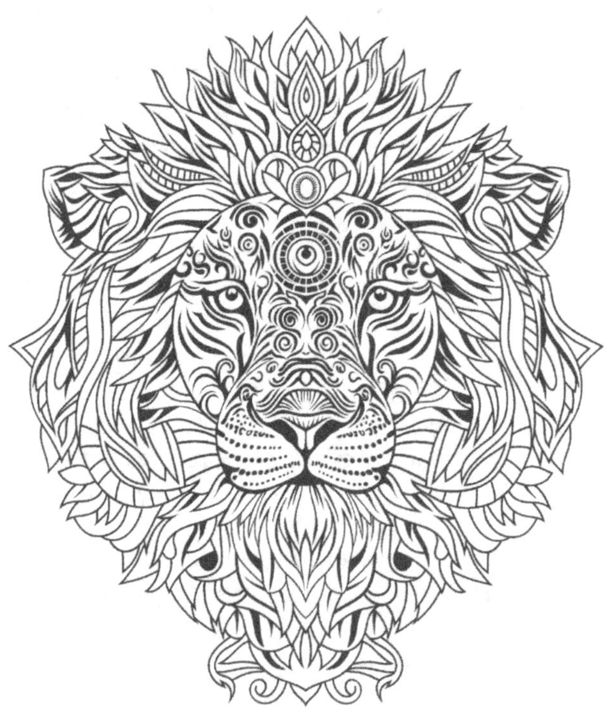

There are only two ways to live your life. One is as though nothing is a miracle. The other is as though everything is a miracle.

- Albert Einstein -

3.16 to 3.26
Siddhis of Jñāna, Sattva, and Manas
Mastery of Wisdom, Spirit, and Mind

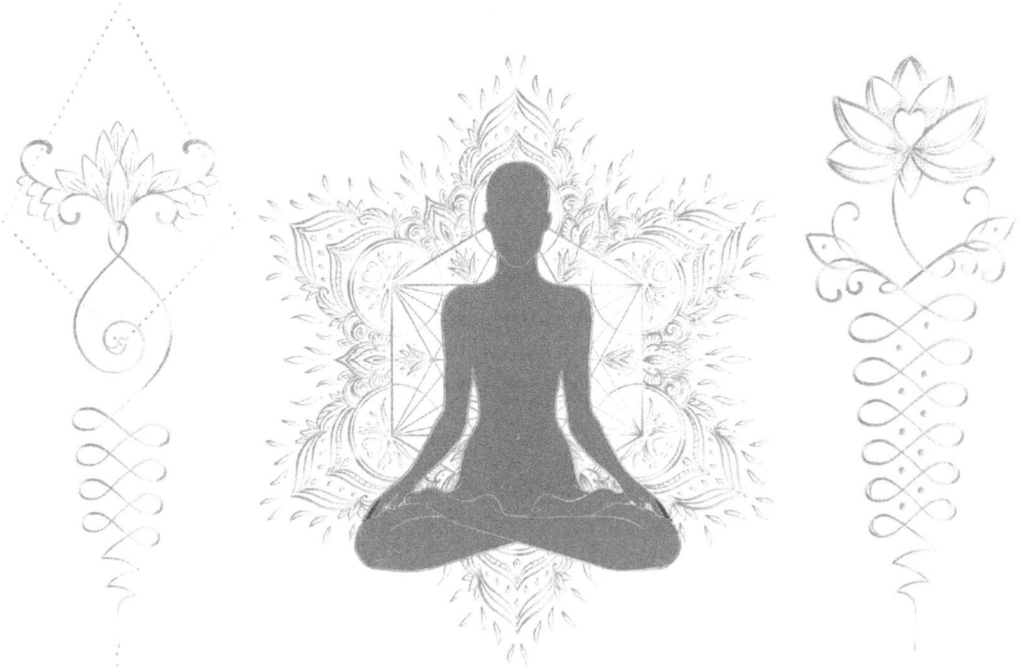

Through the portals of silence the healing sun
of wisdom and peace will shine upon you.
- Paramahansa Yogananda -

3.16

Pariṇāma-traya-saṁyamād atītānāgata-jñānam.

By practicing **saṁyama** on the three transformations (**pariṇāmas**), the yogi gains knowledge (**jñāna**), of past and future events.

Here begins the potential to unlock the mystical gifts of yoga. Through **saṁyama** on the processes of evolution—reflecting on the birth, growth, and eventual dissolution of everything in the natural world (sūtra 3.13)—the yogi accesses **jñāna,** higher knowledge that transcends the constraints of time itself.

Consider the evolution of a rose bush, from the delicate buds of spring to the immense blooms of summer and the gradual fall of the petals back to the earth in the winter, only to begin again the next spring. The rose bush doesn't cling to a withered petal or fear the arrival of winter. Like all growth in nature, it surrenders to its natural rhythm, reminding us that we too can flow freely through the cycles of our own existence.

As we meditate on the past, present, and future, we unlock the gift of enhanced perception and understanding and free our minds from the confines of time. Through **saṁyama** on the three transformations, we untangle ourselves from the shackles of the past and future, creating a tranquil space to drop the weight of old troubles and shed the anxiety of potential future stress.

Consider challenging passages of your own life—the death of a loved one, a career change, divorce, or sudden illness. Just as the rose bush gradually transitions through the seasons, by embracing faith through life's changes, we too rebloom as we wisely surrender to the natural flow of life.

3.17

*Śabdārtha **pratyayānām** itaretarādhyāsāt saṁkarastatpravibhāga samyamāt **sarva** bhūta ruta **jñāna**ṁ.*

Knowledge (**jñāna**) is gained by practicing **samyama** on the words exchanged with others, their meaning, and their underlying concepts (**pratyaya**), enabling deep communication with all (**sarva**).

The words we exchange are essential, but they can also present obstacles. Even speaking the same language, the nuances of personal expression lead to misinterpretation and misunderstanding. Through **samyama** on the duality of language, we grow more self-aware in our communication as we consciously consider how we process others' words and express our own.

Recall a time when you misinterpreted the details of an interaction with a loved one, ruminating over it again and again in your mind, leading to feelings of hurt or resentment. Perhaps a casual remark felt insensitive, however upon reflection, you discovered that the comment was not directed at you, but at their own challenges.

As we empty the mind through meditation, our thoughts become clear, allowing us to better process, interpret, and critically discern the layers of expression beneath our words and the words of others. A practiced yogi not only understands their friends' words without judgment, but also begins to use words more judiciously—limiting those that are unnecessary and carefully choosing what is important.

Through the gift of heightened understanding, we become less reactive, our empathy expands, our communication deepens and all of our relationships improve.

3.18

Saṁskārasākṣātkaraṇāt pūrvajātijñānam.

By practicing **saṁyama** on past impressions (**saṁskāras**), the yogi gains knowledge (**jñāna**) of previous births.

As we continue to refine our perception, we start to see ourselves at the subtlest level. Latent impressions (**saṁskāras**) surface revealing past events, actions, and versions of ourselves. Through **saṁyama**, we gain the ability to confront the marks left upon us by our previous selves. This, of course, does not happen all at once. It is a gradual process of self-unfoldment that awakens the opportunity to heal, forgive and grow.

*Return to your mat to practice **saṁyama** on your **saṁskāras**. As memories from the past surface, sit with the emotions that arise. Don't analyze, resolve, or control the emotions; simply observe how they feel in your body.*

Whatever emotions surface—anxiety, fear, disappointment, grief—let them flow through you. Give these emotions to your breath and notice how they manifest in your body. Let your breath turn these emotions into a gust of positive energy. Envision these oscillating forms (vikṣepa) shifting into something beautiful, like a flower, or the ebb and flow of a wave at the ocean's shore. Let them transform into whatever brings you peace.

Each time an emotion arises, continue to transform it into your positive image. Now, feel the healing sweetness of the present moment and begin to move forward in a space of self-compassion, forgiveness and boundless love.

Through this practice, we begin to embrace the entirety of our personal history, and maybe even past lives. The possibilities are infinite as we continue to self-unfold.

3.19

*Pratyayasya para-citta-**jñānam**.*

[Through *saṁyama*] knowledge (*jñāna*) from another's mind stuff (**pratyaya**) is obtained.

3.20

Na ca tat sālambanam tasyāviṣayī bhūtatvāt.

The physical objects themselves are not included with the divine gift of knowledge.

We've all had moments when it felt like someone could read our minds, perhaps it was with a guru, a shaman, or an insightful friend. Through *saṁyama*, we awaken our natural intuition, enabling us to better recognize the thoughts and feelings of others.

In the vibratory hum of universal connection, subtler levels of perception arise. By cultivating awareness, we foster insight rather than ignorance, reaching a level of discernment where it feels like we can intuitively understand another's thoughts.

This gift, however, has its limits. Patanjali is quick to caution us that, while our skills of perception may be so sharp that we can read minds, we should not assume that we possess mastery or control over another's thoughts. Thank goodness for this because if our minds were filled with others' thoughts, life would be very challenging!

3.21

*Kāya-rūpa-**saṁyamā**t tad-grāhya-śakti-stambhe
cakṣuḥ**prakāśā**saṁprayoge'ntardhānam.*

By **saṁyama** on the body, the yogi can harness the power of invisibility. This is achieved through reflection on the physical form, shadow, light (**prakāśā**), and the eyes.

3.22

Etena śabdādyantardhānam uktam.

The faculties of sound, touch, and taste, etc. can disappear.

3.23

*Sopakramam nirupakramam ca karma tat **saṁyamā**d
aparānta **jñāna**m ariṣṭebhyo vā.*

Through **saṁyama** on **karma,** the yogi gains **jñāna** on time of death.

While these *siddhis* may stretch into unknown territory, contemplating the natural marvels of the world may help us to see the infinite possibilities of the human mind. Phenomena like the migration of monarch butterflies across thousands of miles, the intricate patterns of snowflakes, the formation of rainbows, the stunning colors of a sunset, and the changing of the seasons serve as a testament to the underlying complexity and magic within the natural world. Similarly, through extraordinary practice, remarkable feats become possible *within ourselves.*

The Puranas, the classical collections of Hindu legends and folktales, recount countless stories of the mystical, superhero-like powers of the *rishis.* Legends speak of sages who, through profound meditation and unwavering devotion, gained the ability to communicate with animals, calm storms, bring the dead back to life, heal the wounded with a touch, and conquer evil with the flash of a hand. The Siddhi *Sūtras* too describe some remarkable grand feats that may need to wait for the next lifetime, but we unquestionably encounter miracles and supernatural perception in this reality as our practice deepens.

Students have reported improved vision and heightened senses, sometimes witnessing an aura of color surrounding the body or the complete disappearance of sensory stimulus. Some, too, healed from conditions, both physical and mental.

Through **saṁyama** practice, we are all drawn to deeper layers of meaning and discoveries beyond the surface of things. Invisibility, for instance, reflects more than bodily disappearance. It recognizes the big shift in perception that meditative absorption bestows—the divine power to recognize the true light of all things.

3.24

Maitryādiṣu balāni

By *saṁyama* on friendliness (**maitrī**) powerful friendships are attained.

In a world where connections are often sought through digital networks and online searches, the blend of *saṁyama* with *abhyāsa-vairāgya*—embracing consistency and a healthy level of attachment—guides the mind beyond external dependencies. With practice, the yogi not only deepens their connection with others, but also discovers the boundless power of their own heart to let go and allow love to unfold naturally.

For some, friendliness comes easy, and for others, it takes practice. On our journey towards *samādhi*, we met the Four Keys to Happiness: **maitrī**, *karuṇā*, *muditā*, and *upekṣā* (sūtra 1.33). We nourished our friendships through *dhyāna* on friendliness, compassion, joy and equanimity.

As our capacity for meditative absorption intensifies, we realize that our source of love and friendship resides within, and our external quest for love diminishes. Now, anchored in self-love, self-compassion, and self-understanding, we become deeply connected with divine consciousness.

Through our *saṁyama*, we discover that the relationships we have with others are actually a reflection of the vibration we emanate outward from within ourselves. In the awakening of this truth, our friendships thrive. The yogi embraces the collective consciousness, viewing every individual as a reflection of life itself. Barriers no longer divide, and harmony with all abides.

Hanuman, celebrated for his unwavering dedication and loyalty to Lord Rama, exemplifies the true essence of deep friendship and devotion. Mantras to the monkey God Hanuman are repeated to invoke these virtues. Just as Hanuman's devotion to

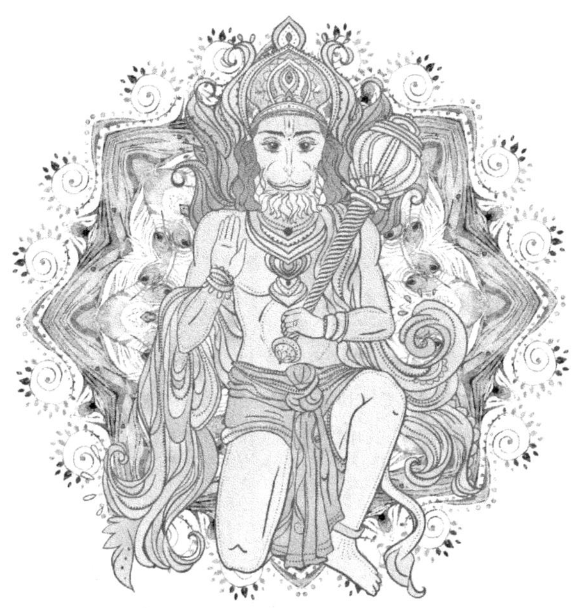

Rama was boundless, by emulating Hanuman's noble qualities and developing our practice of *saṁyama*, we nurture meaningful connections and enduring friendships.

Repeat the following hanuman *bija* mantra inspiring strength and devotion:

Om Ham Hanumate Namah

Invoke the power of **maitrī** as you listen to Hanuman Bolo by Janin Devi and Andre Maris (duet) and full orchestra *with Dj Drez and Janet Stone. (Scan QR code)*

3.25
*Baleṣu **hasti**-balādīni*

By **saṁyama** on the strength of an elephant (**hasti**) great fortitude is attained.

Perhaps you're familiar with the saying "where your attention goes, energy flows." On whatever it is that we practice **saṁyama**, or in whatever it is that we become absorbed in, shapes our experience and personal growth.

Through **saṁyama** on our inner power, we build mammoth resilience. We generate vigor, like the strength of an elephant, to express our personal potential. This powerful fortitude underlies our ability to overcome obstacles with courage and fearlessness.

The elephant carries deep symbolism within Indian culture and yoga philosophy. Ganesha, the elephant-headed god, embodies a fusion of human and elephant attributes. Ganesha's large and perceptive ears inspire us to listen closely to our inner truth. The elephant's tranquil manner reminds us that the quieter we become, the better we perceive the deep wisdom which resides within. By attracting the energy and personifying the disposition of Ganesha, we break through our barriers with a newfound and unwavering strength.

Find a mindful seat and sit with Ganesha. You may use this picture, a statue, or imagine a real elephant in nature. Place your hands on your solar plexus at the front of the ribcage and take a few deep breaths. As you breathe in, visualize drawing in the strength and resilience of an elephant, and allow it to radiate through your core.

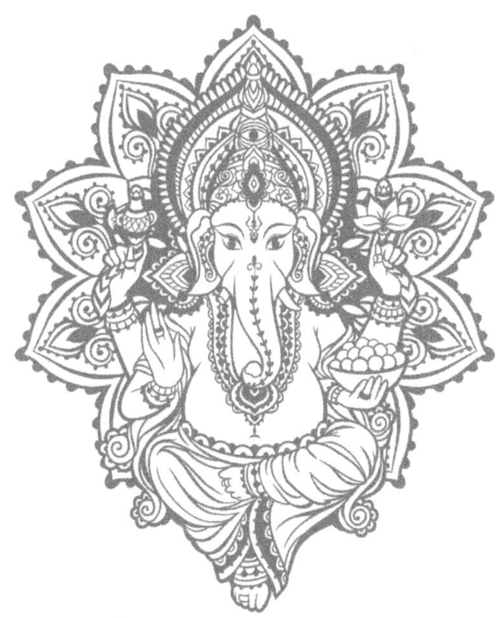

Through japa repeat the Ganapataye mantra (Ganapataye refers to Ganesha) until inner fortitude lights up your being.

Om Gam Ganapataye Namaha, Om Gam Ganapataye Namaha, Om Gam Ganapataye Namaha

Om, Praise to Lord Ganesha, wipe away my negativity, remove my obstacles so that I stand strong in my personal power.

Continue with the *Ganapataye mantra*, stoking your inner strength. Build your core strength with *Power Yoga, Strong Core,* by Dig Yoga. (*Scan QR code*)

3.26

Pravṛttyāloka-nyāsāt sūkṣma-vyavahita-viprakṛṣta-jñānam.

By *saṃyama* on the light within (*āloka*), one gains knowledge (*jñāna*) of subtle (*sūkṣma*), concealed objects.

In Sūtra 3.5, we learned of **prajñālokḥ**, the spark of brilliance within each of us that illuminates and unveils the subtleties and secrets of our incredible world. This **āloka** is our reservoir of *sattva,* the wise, clarifying energy that empowers *siddhās* to bring concealed truths to light.

Enlightenment is fueled by careful study beyond the surface of things to grasp the subtle and hidden aspects of reality. Like a lamp that dispels darkness, *saṃyama* on **āloka** allows us to see what others cannot. Through the exploration of this subtle sense, things that were once concealed to us are now revealed.

Sense your own brilliance by finding a comfortable place, and lying down in savasana. Begin to visualize your skin as a container for your radiant **āloka***. With each breath in, feel this light expanding beyond the boundaries of your skin, filling the room around you with a luminous glow. Then, envision this light expanding further, beyond the walls, embracing your whole community with its warmth and brilliance.*

Extend this light to touch every living being. Now continue, without limitation, beyond to the vastness of the universe. Feel the oneness with the cosmos and the insight revealed. Sense the knowledge far removed from your present sense of being. Sense the universe within you and let the secrets of divine knowledge unfold.

Recognize the infinite light and knowledge which resides within you with this meditation, *You Are the Cosmos!* by Great Meditation. (*Scan QR code*)

3.27 to 3.29
Siddhis
On the Miracles of the Universe

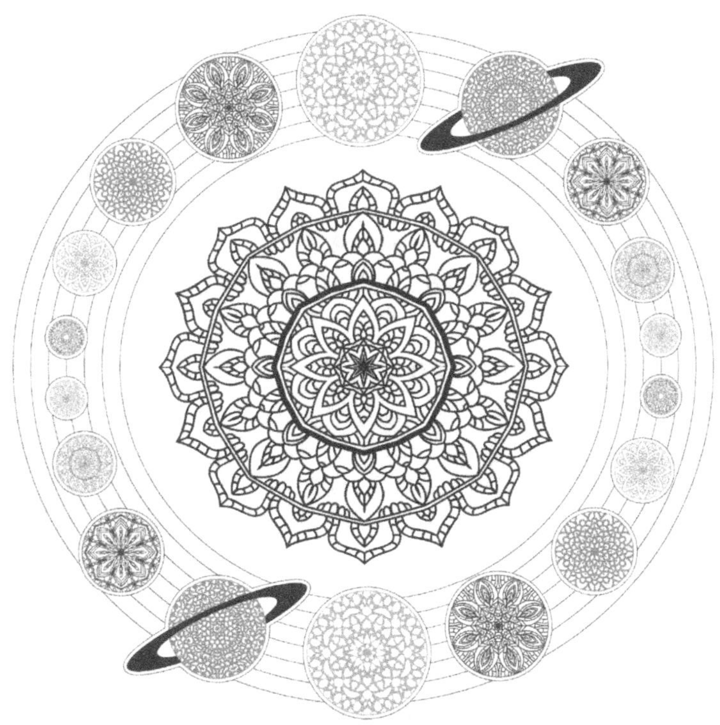

3.27

*Bhuvana-**jñānam** sūrye samyamāt.*

By **samyama** on the sun (**sūrye**) arises wisdom of the realms beyond the solar system.

3.28

*Candre tārā-vyūha-**jñānam**.*

[By **samyama**] on the moon (**candre**) comes **jñāna** on the arrangement of the stars.

3.29

*Dhruve tad-gati-**jñānam**.*

[By **samyama**] on the north star brings **jñāna** of the movement of the stars.

Before scientific tools emerged, classical yoga philosophers observed the universe. A glimpse of their galactic knowledge can be found in the *Vedas*, one of the oldest Indian texts dating back to around 600 BC. Within these ancient scriptures, the *rishis* described remarkable astronomical insights, calculating facts with astonishing accuracy, all without the aid of modern instruments like telescopes[3]. It is believed that their deep understanding arose from the practice of *saṃyama* on the sun, which was aided by focusing on the *surya nāḍī* or *suṣumṇa nāḍī*–the central energy channel running along the spinal column. This practice enabled them to connect with and gain insights into the structure of the universe, the arrangement of stars in galaxies, and the celestial movements that govern our cosmos.

Saṃyama on the sun encompasses rituals and practices aimed at harnessing this great cosmic energy. One such ritual is to focus on the third eye, which is considered the seat of the sun. Another practice is the daily chanting of the Gayatri Mantra, a hymn to the sun god **sūrya**. In Hindu mythology, **sūrya** is depicted as a powerful figure, steering a celestial chariot drawn by seven white horses across the sky. These ancient yogic practices and traditions also gave rise to the Sun Salutations, *Sūrya Namaskāra*, a series of postures and movements still practiced today.

Repeat the Gayatri Mantra, often recited 108 times by devotees in India each morning just before sunrise.

Oṃ bhūḥ bhuvaḥ svaḥ tat savitur vareṇyaṃ bhargo devasya dhīmahi dhiyo yo naḥ pracodayāt

I am light, guiding my way home, I am light the essence of my soul.

The mantra invokes the energy and wisdom of the sun–a testament to Vedic wisdom and its cosmic insights. (*Scan QR code*)

3.30-3.39
Siddhis of the Inner Channels

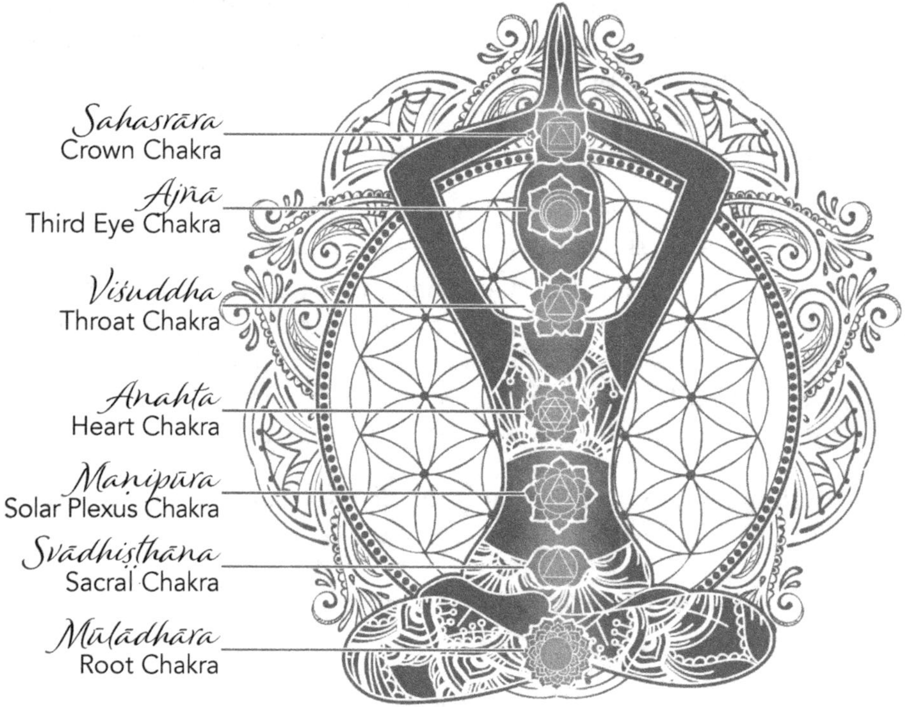

Before we unwrap the gifts of the *siddhis*, let's turn our focus inward to the world of the subtle body known as the chakra system. Yoga philosophy shares seven main chakras or wheels of energy, that extend out from the *suṣumṇa* (sushumna) channel, the main energy channel that runs along the spinal column.

Yoga acts as the spark that awakens these dormant centers. Think of them as powerhouses, waiting to be activated to ignite our greatest potential. The higher we explore the chakras, which ascend from the base of the spine to the crown of the skull, the higher the frequencies and vibrations that attune our being. This is also referred to as Kundalini rising.

Working on any one chakra will affect the entire system of chakras. As *prana* flows freely through these energy channels, we express the highest potential of each vortex. When we commit to understanding and mastering the higher vibrations, we transcend imbalances and our spirit soars.

Before we continue with Patanjali's exploration of the *chakras* (Patanjali refers to them as *nadis*) let us first define the seven main energy centers.

The journey through these vortexes begins at *mūlādhāra* chakra, located at the base of the spine. Here lies our sense of stability, security, and connection to the earth. As this feeling of grounding blossoms, unwavering confidence and courage ensues.

Moving upwards to the lower pelvic region is *svādhiṣṭhāna*, the sacral chakra, the center of innovation, passion, and the water element. When activated, it unleashes a deep sense of emotional well-being, creative energy and sensual vitality.

Maṇipūra, the solar plexus chakra, sits just above the navel, radiating personal power and will. Activation of *maṇipūra* empowers us to harness our inner fire, which imparts confidence, drive, and a balanced sense of self.

Venturing higher is *anahata*, the heart chakra, at the center of the chest, where the element of air resides. This energy center is the hub of love, empathy, and connection. An awakened heart chakra leads to boundless compassion, harmonious relationships, and the ability to embrace both ourselves and others unconditionally.

Progressing further we come to *viśuddha*, the throat chakra, nestled in the front of the neck. The element at this *chakra* is space. *Viśuddha* symbolizes clear communication and self-expression. Activating this center empowers us to speak our truth, liberating our authentic voice and fostering genuine interactions.

Ajñā, the third eye chakra, is located between the eyebrows and enables us to see beyond the surface. *Ajñā* opens the gateway to insight, connecting us to our inner wellspring of wisdom, which includes access to heightened intuition and a deepened connection with our highest Self.

Lastly, the *sahasrāra* or crown chakra is situated at the top of the head. It signifies enlightenment and the spiritual connection we experience outside the boundaries of our minds. Activation aligns us with universal consciousness, expanding our awareness beyond our individual sense of being.

Feel the somatic connection with each chakra as you place your hands at the desired energetic center. Repeat the associated mantra, allowing its spirit to infuse your breath. Sense the prana circulating through the surrounding area of the body aligning with the focused chakra.

Mūlādhāra (pelvic floor): *I am always safe, rooted and grounded from the center of my being.*

Svādhiṣṭhāna (below the naval): *I flow with the rhythm of life.*

Maṇipūra (solar plexus): *I stand in my personal power.*

Anahata (heart): *I open my heart to all with unconditional love.*

Viśuddha (throat): *I follow and speak my truth.*

Ājñā (third eye): *I follow my wisdom the path of truth.*

Sahasrāra (crown of the head): *A greater power connects me to all that I do.*

Explore the awakening of the subtle body with this chakra practice by Yoga Awakening with Sue. (*Scan QR code*)

(*For more information on each chakra see Appendix E: Chakra Outline, page 272.*)

3.30
Nābhi-cakre kāya-vyūha-jñānam.

Saṁyama on the navel (**nābhi**) plexus brings knowledge (**jñāna**) of the anatomy of the body.

Spiraling upwards from the dense lower chakras to the higher realms of awakening, Patanjali undertakes a bodily exploration starting from the **nābhi** chakra. Ancient sages believed it to be the root of the *nāḍīs*. It is similar to the modern equivalent of the *maṇipūra* chakra.

Located at the navel or solar plexus, **nābhi** chakra is the cradle of our existence. It is our primal site of energy, where we were once nurtured within the womb. When we direct our attention to *maṇipūra* chakra, we not only gain insight into the mechanics of the physical body, but also tap into our wellspring of inner fortitude and self-confidence.

Practices involving *nābhi* chakra include *uḍḍīyana bandha*. This *bandha* technique involves contracting the abdominal muscles, drawing the navel inward and upward towards the spine, and holding the breath for a few moments. *Uḍḍīyana bandha* is one of the four sacred locks used to direct the flow of energy and enhance physical and energetic alignment. The other *bandhas* are *mūla*, *jālandhara*, and *mahā*.

Bring your awareness to the solar plexus by placing your hands at the base of the rib cage. Take a deep inhale through the nose. Feel the space grow between the ribs, and hold this expansion. Exhale through the mouth with pursed lips, as if blowing through a straw. Inhale "inspiration," exhale, with pursed lips "elimination". Feel your vitality and positive energy expand outward like spokes of a wheel, unfolding from this hub of strength.

Join Jessica Heslop in this practice for the *maṇipūra* chakra. (*Scan QR code*)

3.31

Kaṇṭha-kūpe kṣut-pipāsā-nivṛttiḥ.

Saṁyama on the throat (**kantha**) brings the cessation of hunger and thirst.

3.32

Kūrma-nāḍyām sthairyaṁ.

Through *saṁyama* on the tortoise nadi (**kūrmanāḍyā**), a still meditative posture is achieved.

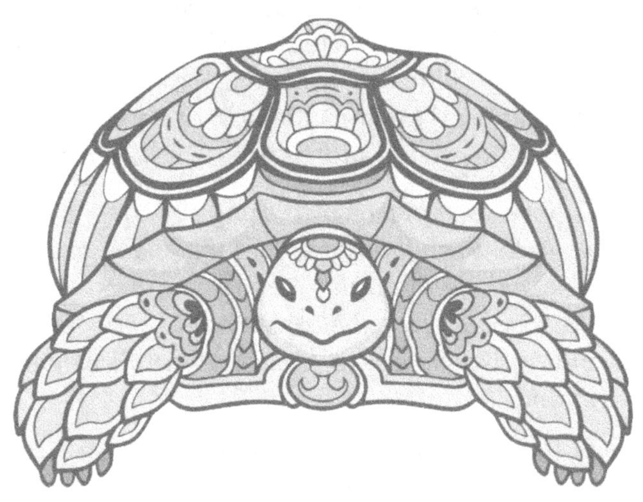

Just like the tortoise who retreats into its shell for protection, *saṁyama* on the tortoise *nāḍī* instills fearlessness and unwavering strength. Both the throat and the tortoise *nāḍī* (**kūrma-nāḍyā**) are intimately connected to the *viśuddha* chakra.

The tortoise *nāḍī* is located in the chest, one inch below where the collar bones meet. By focusing our attention on our bony sternum, we fortify our outer layer of steadfastness. When *prana* flows freely through this chakra, we gain the ability to speak our truth with clarity and confidence.

Saṁyama on the throat can also lead to the cessation of hunger and thirst. While this may initially appear impossible, studies[4] suggest that advanced meditators can influence their autonomic nervous system regulating bodily functions like heart rate, digestion, and respiratory rate. Practicing postures which support throat opening such as fish pose can also help to awaken this energy area.

Find a comfortable seated position, with a straight spine and shoulders relaxed. Take a few deep breaths to center yourself. Direct your awareness to the tortoise nāḍī located just below where the collar bones meet. Gently place your fingertips on this area, tuning into the subtle sensations beneath your touch.

Connect with the tortoise nāḍī, and visualize your rib cage as your guarding armor, like the sturdy shell of a turtle. Envision the shield surrounding your heart center as a sanctuary of security and stability. With each breath, allow your protective shell to become more vivid and present, letting it envelope your being with strength and power.

Continue reinforcing your inner strength and practice *saṁyama* on the tortoise *nāḍī* with *Kurma Nadi: The Tortoise Meditation. (Scan QR code)*

3.33

Mūrdha-jyotiṣi siddha-darśanaṁ.

Focusing on the light (**jyoti**) at the crown of the head, visions of **siddhas,** perfected beings, are revealed.

The *sahasrāra* chakra, extending from the crown of the skull, is the culmination of our spiritual ascent. When activated, this highest point of the chakra system is sometimes referred to as kundalini awakening.

By directing our attention to the inner light at this sacred center we unlock the potential for extraordinary experiences. These include visions of *siddhas*—enlightened beings who have transcended the limitations of the physical realm or wisdom arising from our revered *gurus* from the past. Through this focused connection with the higher chakras, our *shakti*, our inner wellspring of power, amplifies, forging a link to higher planes of consciousness.

Close your eyes and take a few deep breaths. Visualize the sahasrāra chakra as a brilliant white lotus at the crown of your head, its expanse like a thousand white petals radiating light in all directions. Sense the brilliance emanating out from the center of this lotus, allowing it to grow brighter with each breath. Envision this light extending from the skull out to the cosmos.

Bring forth those of your past whose wisdom shines bright within you. Maybe a deceased family member, friend, spiritual teacher or even an animal. Feel the connection to their spirit and the higher realms of consciousness. Sit here embodied in the presence of their wisdom, letting this illumination carry you throughout your day.

Tap into your awareness of the vastness of the universe focusing on the Third Eye (*ajna chakra*) and crown chakra with this meditation by Zia - Manifesto Meditations. (*Scan QR code*)

3.34
*Prātibhād vā **sarvaṁ***

Through intuition comes all (**sarva**) [knowledge].

As our *shakti* rises extraordinary insight is revealed. By focusing on the throat, third eye, and crown of the head, we begin to open the door to divine intuition, the innate knowledge that transcends the boundaries of logic and sensory perception. This intuition, extends beyond what can be learned through conventional means and analytical thinking. Patanjali reminds us that the most profound insights arise from within.

Think of those moments when knowledge seemed to innately flow through you. Yoga instructors often experience this phenomenon when teaching. While explanations of philosophy and other insights may not come readily in everyday life, through concentration and connection with our intuition, a wealth of understanding effortlessly unfurls.

Continue to take time each day to create a sanctuary for stillness and inner listening.

Sit comfortably with your spine straight, close your eyes, and take a deep breath. Bring your awareness to your throat, feeling the energy center there, and breathe deeply. Move your focus to your third eye, in the middle of your forehead, and soften into the insight unfolding. Continue to bring your awareness from the throat to the third eye and the third eye back to the throat. Repeat internally, "I follow and speak my truth, I follow my intuition the path of truth." Finally, direct your attention to the crown of your head, visualizing a gentle light pouring in. Feel this light filling you with infinite wisdom and intuitive knowledge. Trust in this inner guidance, knowing it transcends ordinary understanding. Remain in stillness, letting this divine insight flow through you effortlessly.

3.35

*Hṛdaye **citta**-saṁvit*

[*Saṁyama* on] the heart brings knowledge of the **citta.**

Moving to the seat of cosmic consciousness, we shift downward to focus on the heart chakra. While the heart chakra might be positioned "lower," it reaches "higher" in terms of its ability to connect with universal understanding. The *anahata* chakra represents the bridge between the physical and spiritual realms.

By *saṁyama* on the heart, we are reminded that we must transcend the limitations of the intellect to access the vast and supreme insights that lie beyond rational understanding. It is through this gateway that the energies of love and compassion pass through us and move onwards to all of humanity.

With hands in prayer at the front of the chest, bring your awareness to anahata chakra. Imagine your heart center as a radiant lotus flower. Envision your blossoming lotus in a color that resonates with the essence of your being. Then, fully embody your lotus by bringing your pinkie fingers and thumbs together in padma mudra.

Let your palms float in front of your heart, fingers continuing to spread open and unfurl. Feel the petals unfold within you, feel the deep wisdom unraveling with each breath. As you inhale and exhale, float your padma mudra towards your third eye, then lower the hands back towards the heart. Repeat this practice until you sense your insight in full bloom.

Continue focusing on the heart chakra with the following meditation.
 (Scan QR code)

3.36

Sattva-puruṣayor atyantāsaṁkīrṇayoḥ **pratyayāviśeṣo bhogaḥ** parārthāt svārtha-**saṁyamāt puruṣa-jñānam**.

Even a clear *citta* is different from **puruṣa**. Although knowledge exists for the sake of **puruṣa,** when there is no distinction of this difference, individual awareness misidentifies with experiences and perceptions. With **saṁyama** on **puruṣa** comes an understanding of this distinction.

In the awakening of our greatest potential, we become firmly anchored in our *sattvic* foundation of tranquility, balance, and illumination. Through our *saṁyama* on *puruṣa* (the spirit) and *buddhi* (the intellect), we recognize the interplay between eternal consciousness (the Knower), our mental processes (the process of Knowing), and our experience of the external world (the Known).

In daily life, these boundaries easily blur, leading us to forget that we are the spark of the Eternal *ātmān*. We find ourselves caught in a cycle of seeking pleasure (*raga*), avoiding pain (*dvesa*) and attaching ourselves to the external world (**bhoga**). In *saṁyama* on *puruṣa*, we sharpen our ability to discern when we are being driven by *citta-vrttis*, the prakṛtic mind. By continually bringing ourselves back to pure awareness, we understand that our intellect, in its finite awareness, perceives the world through a limited filter.

*Find a comfortable space, close your eyes and focus on your breath. Shift your attention inward, observing your thoughts and sensations. Center on the space of pure awareness. Return to the question: Who am I? Meditate on your true essence, letting go of attachment to your thoughts, beliefs and ideas. Notice the distinction between that which is fluctuating and that which remains constant, and observe what unfolds for you. Dive deeper into eternal joy and sit with the Knower–**puruṣa**. Hold this understanding in the present moment to foster harmony amidst the intricate dance of collective consciousness, the individual mind, and our present perception of the external world.*

3.37

*Taṭ **prātibha** śrāvaṇa vedanādarśāsvāda vārtā jāyante.*

From this arises intuition (**prātibha**) as well as supernatural hearing, touch, vision, taste, and smell.

As insight and intuition thrive through *saṁyama on **puruṣa***, our senses hum at a higher vibration. Mastery of this *siddhi*–supernatural sensory receptors–is extraordinary, revealing an enhanced perception of our relative world.

As our mind sharpens, we perceive with greater clarity. Where once we might have overlooked the vibrant colors of a beautiful sunrise or a blooming garden, the details of life are now strikingly vivid. Through our heightened lens of **prātibha** we embrace each moment with wonder and experience the full richness of life in every sense.

Today, focus on being fully present with your senses. Begin by inhaling deeply, attuning your sense of smell to the subtle aromas that linger in the air. Feel the textures and temperatures on your skin, and ground your awareness in the present moment. Let your eyes wander, and taste the vivid colors and shapes of your immediate environment. Listen intently to the nuances of life–a distant melody, the gentle rustle of leaves, or the soothing song of nature. Let the subtleties of the present touch your spirit.

As you deepen your breath, visualize a soft, radiant light encircling you, bringing a sense of peace and tranquility. With each inhale, draw in this healing light, and with each exhale, release any tension or stress. Embrace the present moment fully and appreciate the beauty that unfolds in each breath and sensation. Engage with your loved ones and even those new to you with a mindful presence, listening intently and cherishing the uniqueness of each interaction.

Continue this practice with *5 Senses Guided Imagery*. (*Scan QR code*)

3.38

*Te samādhāvupasargā vyutthāne **siddhayḥ**.*

These extraordinary senses are accomplishments (**siddhis**) to the mind but hinder the attainment of **samādhi**.

Patanjali takes pause here to remind us that, while the attainment of extraordinary senses is an accomplishment, these experiences can create obstacles along the path to our ultimate goal. He cautions us not to develop attachment to the *siddhis*, otherwise, our cravings for these milestones could prevent us from reaching *samādhi*.

Even though the **siddhis** are enticing, seeking them shifts our focus away from connecting with our *ātmān*. When any specific element—negative or positive—takes precedence over the goal of divine awareness, it disrupts our inner balance and harmony. To continue on our path we must move beyond the confines of the mind and enter the limitless expanse of our spiritual being.

Progress is gained on the path when a yogi practices with his or her whole heart. With sincerity and the release of the desire for outcomes true Freedom flourishes.

3.39

Bandha-kāraṇa-śaithilyāt pracāra-saṁvedanāc ca cittasya para-śarīrāveśḥ.

By releasing the bind (**bandha**) of the mind (**citta**), and by knowledge of the energy channels within, entering another's body is possible.

As we awaken our energy centers by ascending into the realm of higher consciousness, our wisdom, intuition and compassion expand. With divine knowledge and insight, we gain the ability to step into the emotions and experiences of others. While we may not actually physically enter their bodies, we now carry a deeper sense of empathy, kindness and understanding in all our relationships.

In embracing the joys and struggles of those around us we begin to feel the Oneness of all humanity, recognizing others as a true reflection of ourselves. With an expanded horizon of consciousness, we wholeheartedly accept others' feelings and perceptions of reality, and although different from ours, our now infinite love allows us to create a sacred space where empathy and divine compassion flourish for all.

Continue to clear the energetic centers and sensory pathways by chanting the seed mantras (*bija mantras*) associated with each chakra.

Lam-root, *Vam*-sacral/navel, *Ram*-solar plexus, *Yam*-heart chakra, *Ham*-throat chakra, *Om*-third eye/brow, *Ah*-crown chakra.

Follow along with *Chakra Seed Mantra Meditation*, by 3 Nity Brothers with Gaia Meditation. (Scan *QR code*)

3.40 to 3.45
Siddhis of the Vayus
Mastery of the Inner Winds

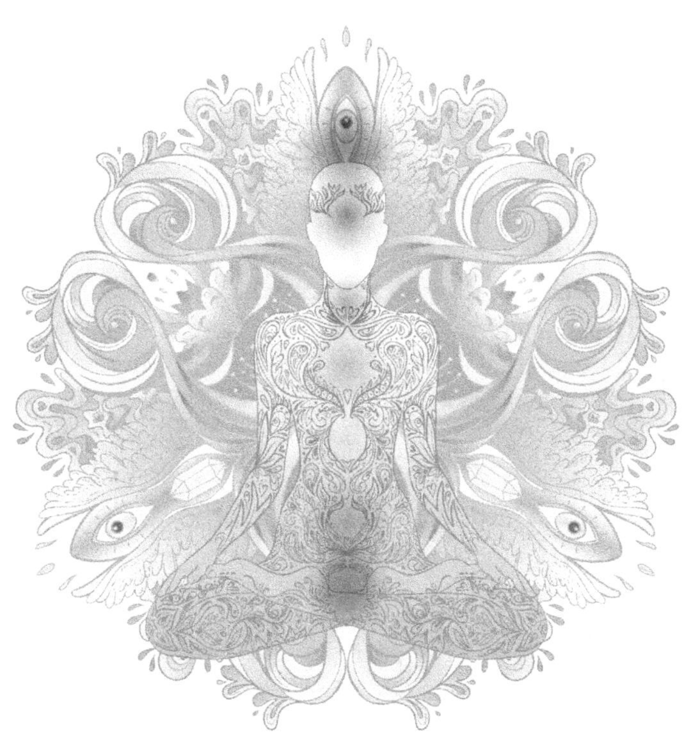

3.40

Udāna*-*jayāj jala-paṅka-kaṇṭakādiṣv asaṅga utkrāntiś ca.

Through mastery over **udāna**, the upward current of *prana*, one can levitate over mud, thorns, and earth.

3.41

Samāna*-*jayāj jvalanaṁ.

By mastery over **samāna**, the equalizing circulation of *prana*, a radiance illuminates the body.

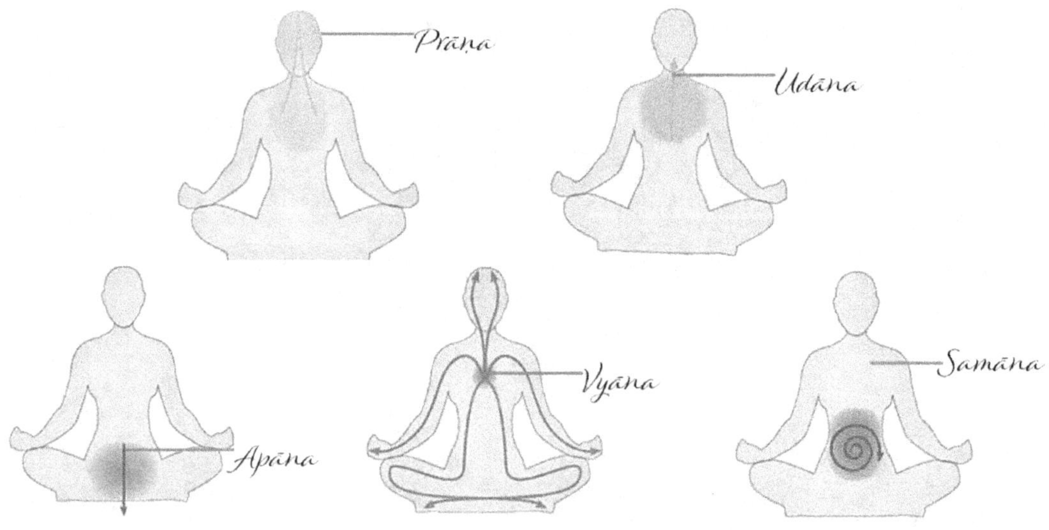

Vayus, the movements of *prāṇa*, are the life force energy that enlivens the body. The five main vayus–*prāṇa*, *apāna*, **samāna**, **udāna**, and *vyāna*–direct the inner symphony of physiological processes that orchestrate our energetic and bodily harmony.

When *saṁyama* is practiced on the *vayus*, hidden pathways within are unlocked granting access to extraordinary abilities. While techniques specific to each *vayu*, such as Kundalini *kriyas*, may not necessarily defy gravity, mastering *udāna*–the upward flow of energy–inspires a lightness of spirit, enabling one to transcend the challenges of life–its mud, thorns, and earthly burdens.

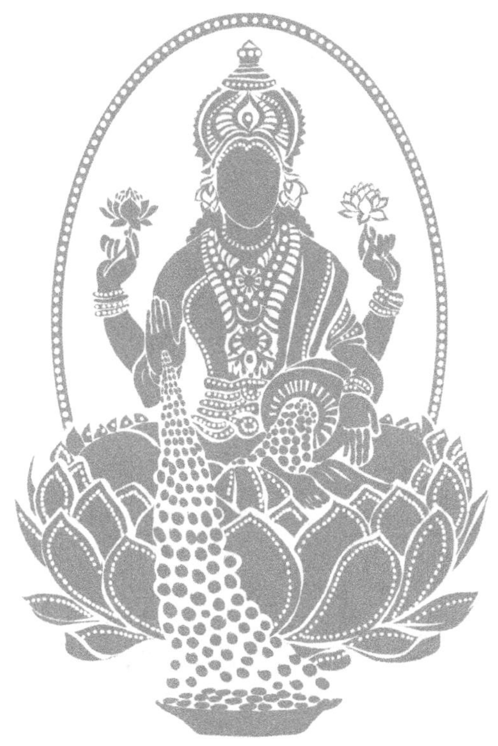

Samāna, the equalizing wind of energy that resides at the navel and abdomen (sūtra 3.41) awakens the fire within. Not only does *samāna* aid in digestion, assimilation, and nutrition, but it also kindles an aura of well-being that projects outwardly. You likely know someone who exudes this radiance, projecting an aura of light and love solely through their presence, without uttering a word.

True levity arises from connecting with and expanding our *ananda*, our blissful lotus of inner radiance. When we tap into our reservoir of inner joy with mantras to Lakshmi, the goddess of abundance and beauty, we connect with the subtle forces behind her goddess energy and, like Lakshmi, glow with a glorious aura.

*Find your mindful seat and attune to the natural rhythm of your breath. Sense the sweet flow of **prāṇa**, the abundance of Lakshmi, moving inwards and up through you. Turn your palms skyward, raise your hands, and enjoy the upward, rising flow of energy.*

*Now, turn your palms downward and lower your hands. Feel the downward and outward flow of apāna vayu. With each exhale, release tension and let negativity melt downwards and away. Place your hands in front of your abdomen, and, without touching the belly, make a circular motion around your navel center. Feel the warm current of Lakshmi circulating around your hands and sense into the flow of **samāna** vayu. Allow these inner winds to balance the fire that harmonizes your internal organs.*

*Shift your focus to **udāna** vayu and the energy that rises from the heart to the head. Juggling hands in front of the throat, sense the uplifting winds that connect the energies of the lower body with the higher planes of consciousness. Hover your hands an inch over the body, and broaden your awareness to vyāna vayu. Sense the winds that circulate the entire body and connect all aspects of your being spreading* *healing energy from center out and fostering unity and coherence through every limb, every organ, and every cell, carrying away any tension or blockages.*

Invoke Lakshmi and awaken the higher realms of Śrī Ānanda to carry the awareness of the balanced flow of the five vayus with you:

Om Shreem Maha Lakshmi Namaha

I invoke the energy of Lakshmi for spiritual and worldly abundance.

Explore the direction and subtleties of the 5 vayus with the following practice and invoke an aura of abundant radiance with this modernized Lakshmi *mantra*, Sam Garrett's, *Lakshmi – I choose to Live in Love. (Scan QR code)*

3.42

*Śrotrākāśayoḥ saṁbandha-**saṁyamād** divyaṁ śrotram.*

By **saṁyama** on the relationship between the organ of the ear and ether, divine hearing is attainable.

3.43

*Kāyākāśayoḥ saṁbandha-**saṁyamāl** laghu-tūla-samāpatteś cākāśa-gamanaṁ.*

By **saṁyama** between the body and ether (**ākāśa**) and the lightness of cotton, traveling through the sky becomes possible.

3.44

*Bahir-akalpitā vṛttir **mahā-videhā** taṭh **prakāśāvaraṇa-kṣayḥ**.*

External awareness ceases when the veil that conceals the light (**prakāśā**) is removed, leading to an out-of-body experience (**mahā videhā**).

As our shakti rises and awakens the flow of our inner winds, we begin to witness states of consciousness beyond the ordinary. Through exploration of different *kriyas*, especially in the practice of Kundalini yoga, our meditation may bring about an out-of-body experience or a feeling of lightness like we could float away. While these occurrences may initially seem miraculous, with deepened perception, we recognize our newfound abilities as transcending the elements of nature.

We have all faced challenging times when we carried the weight of the world on our shoulders, feeling sad or discouraged. In such states our bodies may feel physically heavy—like gravity is pulling us down. Through *kriya* practices that redirect energy upward to the lighter and higher *chakras* and focus on **ākāśa** (ether), we become buoyant, uplifted, happy, and carefree.

The practice of yoga removes the veils that conceal the light (**prakāśā**) of the Self and the emotional heaviness that comes with it. According to a modern scientific view, on an atomic level, our bodies are predominantly composed of space. By drawing our attention from denser to subtler dimensions, the yogi gains an experiential understanding of this paradox, transcending the fundamental building blocks of the material world—earth, water, fire, air, and ether.

Through steady practice, we refine our energies and gain insight into the natural order of things. We start to notice the intricate play of the chakras and the vayus, and awaken subtler realms of reality. In our own journey of transformation, suddenly, defying gravity doesn't seem like such a far-fetched idea.

Neither does a **mahā videhā,** an extraordinary out-of-body experience!

3.45

Sthūla-svarūpa-sūkṣmānvayārthavattva-saṁyamād bhūta-jayḥ.

*By practicing **saṁyama** on the gross (**sthūla**), subtle (**sūkṣmā**), innate characteristics (**svarūpa**), and purpose, mastery over the elements (**bhūta**) is attained.*

Through the steady practice of concentrated meditative absorption, we learn to explore the elements from all perspectives. Whether it be gross (**sthūla**) like earth, or subtle (**sūkṣmā**) like gravity, this practice helps our abilities grow in extraordinary ways. Suddenly, instead of sweating the small stuff, we find new strength in **saṁyama** on the **svarūpa**, the true nature of all things.

As the yogi's practice grows more refined, each chakra and its related element becomes a gateway that unlocks deeper layers within. As each element is addressed through different yogic practices that invoke subtler molecular qualities, the yogi awakens specific energy channels that promote a harmonious flow within the body.

The awakening of the energy centers and the subtle vayus in a literal and profound sense enables the yogi to navigate the realms of both humanity and divinity. When all aspects of the elements (**bhūtas**) are fully considered, the yogi learns to harmonize with the fundamental fabric of reality. Attuned to the subtle energies, the yogi experiences the world not merely through the lens of individuality, but as part of the vast cosmic tapestry.

3.46
The 8 Mystical Siddhis

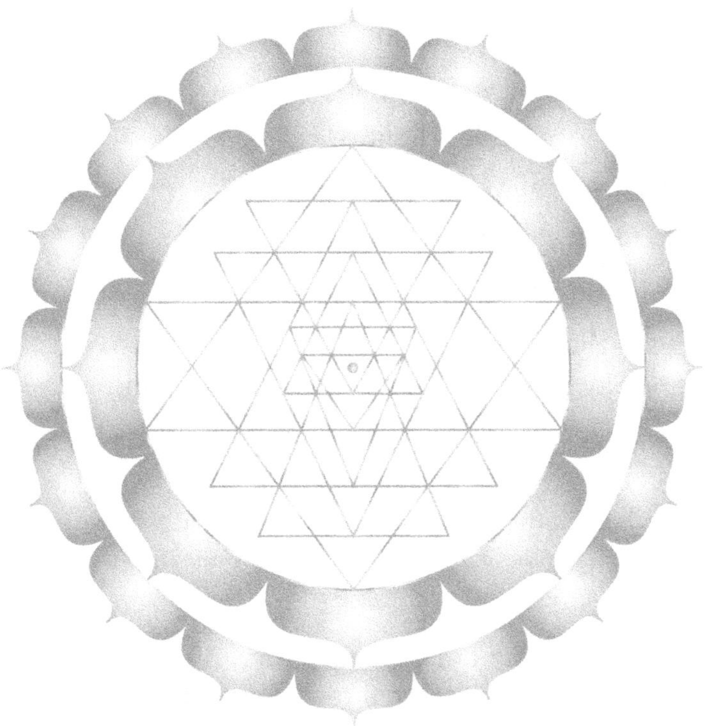

3.46

Tato' ṇimādi-prādurbhāvḥ kāya-saṁpat-tad-dharmānabhighātaś ca.

[By mastery over the bhūtas] the body's limitations can be overcome through development of the eight mystic powers:

1. *Aṇimā* (to become very small)

2. *Mahima* (to become very big)

3. *Laghima* (to become very light)

4. *Garima* (to become very heavy)

5. *Prāpti* (to reach anywhere)

6. *Prākāmya* (to achieve all one's desires)

7. *Iṣṭva* (ability to create anything)

8. *Vaśitva* (ability to command and control everything)

After discovering mastery over the elements and overcoming our personal limitations, a cosmic body emerges as we find release from the shackles of identification with the outer world. By cutting our ties with attaining perfection of our temporary, ever-changing outer shell, we stop identifying with our gross vessel and turn to the mystical.

Think of the significant investment of time, money and stress that we allocate for the outer perfection of the body. When the yogi begins to release the unnecessary, finding more time for **saṁyama**, a pivotal shift occurs. Now the limitless capabilities of the mind and consciousness are unveiled.

3.47 to 3.49
The Qualities of the Siddha
Attaining Perfection and Freedom

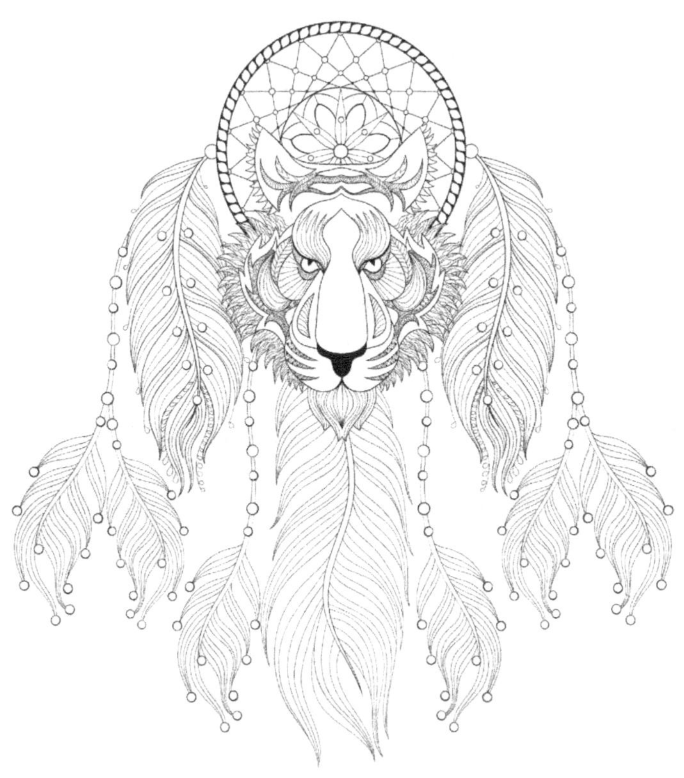

3.47

Rūpa-lāvaṇya-bala-vajra-saṁhananatvāni kāya-saṁpat.

Perfection of the body manifests the qualities of beauty, grace, strength, and the power of a thunderbolt (**vajra**).

Through unwavering *abhyāsa*, the yogi becomes a living embodiment of beauty, grace, and perfection. Like the power of a thunderbolt (*vajra*), the yogi stands strong and invincible. This strength is both physical and dynamic and the yogi possesses a superhuman capacity to overcome any obstacle or challenge.

Even in the face of life's adversities, through *tapas* and *abhyāsa* the yogi gains the ability to reduce or completely remove all mental distress and suffering. Through this transformation, the body is now a sacred vessel for spiritual growth and self-realization. Aligned with divine qualities, the yogi becomes a living testament to the harmonious integration of the physical and spiritual realms.

The Hindu deity Indra, associated with thunder and lightning, (**vajra**) mirrors this invincible strength. Indra wields the *thunderbolt* as a symbol of his indestructible power. Similarly, the yogi, having harnessed the power of yoga, stands firm with an indomitable force.

Indra's strength lies not just in physical might but in his ability to overcome misfortune. Similarly, the yogi's strength goes beyond muscular prowess, encompassing resilience, discipline, and an unyielding capacity to face and conquer life's trials. The yogi stands strong in love and grace instead of fear and darkness.

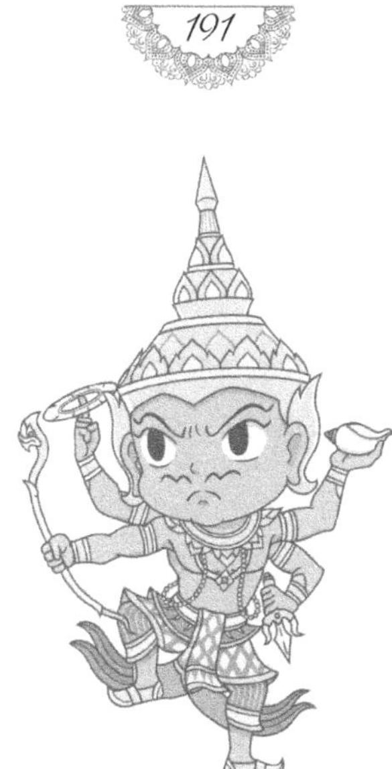

The *vajra*, also known as *dorje* in Tibetan Buddhism is an object holding deep symbolism. Translating to "diamond" or "thunderbolt," it signifies the indestructible and unchanging nature of Enlightenment. Paired with a bell in Tibetan Buddhist rituals, the *vajra* and bell together symbolize the integration of wisdom and compassion, essential for attaining Enlightenment.

Here you can find more information on the vajra or dorje and also its use in sound healing. (*Scan QR code*)

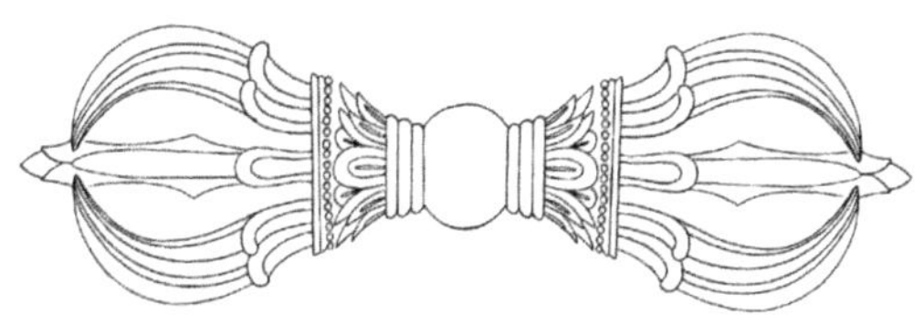

3.48

*Grahaṇa-**svarūpāsmitā**nvayārthavattva-**saṃyamād indriya**-jayaḥ.*

Through the practice of **saṃyama** on the process of perception, the essence of being (**svarūpa**), the ego (**asmitā**), and the nature and purpose [of the *guṇas*], arrives mastery over the senses (**indriyas**).

Now, the *siddha*, the perfected body, is a vessel through which the yogi attains mastery over the sensory realm. Imagine experiencing the world not through the lens of the eyes, ears, nose, tongue, and skin, but beyond their conventional boundaries. **Saṃyama** on the senses enables the yogi to tap into profound realms of divine insight, experiencing subtleties that go unnoticed by ordinary perception.

In our relative world, human senses have limited capabilities. Yet, consider the heightened perception of members of the animal kingdom, such as the acute vision of birds or the ability of bats to navigate through echolocation. Similarly, through the practice of **saṃyama** on the process of perception, we transcend the limits of sensory perception and awaken previously unknown levels of awareness.

As the yogi refines their ability to perceive, the world becomes a canvas of rich and intricate sensations. The rustling leaves, the fragrance of flowers, the sunset—all the workings of nature unfold with new vibrancy. For the evolved yogi, life gains new richness and abundance, and with this heightened awareness the ordinary becomes extraordinary.

3.49

Tato mano-javitvam vikaraṇa-bhāvḥ pradhāna-jayaś ca.

Through mastery, nerve impulses quicken and the mind disconnects from the senses. Complete control over *prakṛti* is achieved.

While we may not have the physical capability to become as small as a mouse or as big as an elephant, our practice grants us many gifts as our true Nature unfolds.

As modern science continues to unravel the mysteries of our universe, yogis believe our inner journey holds the potential for even deeper revelations. Through disciplined *saṁyama* practice, the yogi establishes a profound connection with and mastery over the subtle forces governing the universe.

With the progression, refinement, and harmonization of *prana*, a metamorphosis occurs. Through the awakening of the subtle energies of the chakras and our connection with the movement of the *vayus*, the yogi's cells become supercharged with spiritual vibrations.

As the nerve impulses quicken, we begin to respond with greater efficiency and wisdom. With each breath and every mindful step, the yogi builds discipline, refines the ability to manage energy, and fosters vitality.

Transcend the senses with this practice by Mooji, *Seeing Without Eyes, Knowing Without Mind. (Scan QR code)*

3.50 to 3.52
The End of Worldly Attachment

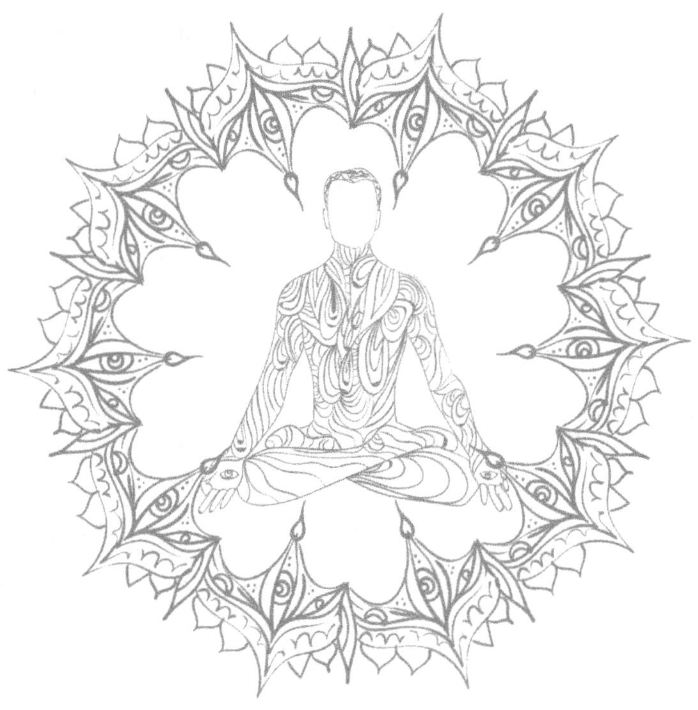

A feeling of aversion or attachment towards something
is your clue that there's work to be done.

- Ram Dass -

3.50

Sattvapuruṣānyatākhyātimātrasya sarvabhāvādhiṣṭhātṛtvam sarvajñātṛtvam ca.

When the difference between the *citta* and **puruṣā** is recognized the yogi obtains omniscience (**sarva-jñātṛtvam**) and unlimited power.

Whether we attain superpowers or not, the true path is discovering our higher Self, the *ātmān*. The *ātmān* is that spark of **puruṣā** within each of us, the eternal Self that is unchanging within every human being.

Through the process of self-unfoldment, the inner space opens to higher realms of consciousness. Now there is complete understanding between what is finite and what is infinite. *Iśvara*, the state of omnipotence and omniscience (**sarva-jñātṛtvam**), is now functioning within. The *yogi* has transformed into a *siddha,* a powerhouse of all-knowingness and limitless strength.

It is extraordinary to contemplate the immense potential that is possible on this journey. The capacity of acquiring superhuman abilities is extreme. However, regardless of whether these extraordinary powers are attained or not, with practice, we learn that our genuine strength lies within the depths of our own being. By first embracing the purity of **sattva** and then merging with the eternal source of **puruṣā**, the yogi stumbles into the realm of true miracles.

3.51

*Tad-**vairāgyā**d api doṣa-**bīja**-kṣaye **kaivalyam**.*

By non-attachment (**vairāgyā**) to the outcome of superpowers, the seeds (**bīja**) of worldly attachment are destroyed, and the yogi finds supreme liberation (**kaivalya**).

3.52

*Sthānyupanimantraṇe saṅga-**smayā**karaṇam punar-aniṣṭa-prasaṅgāt.*

There should be no pride (**smayā**) in our accomplishments, even when praised by those in high places.

No matter how miraculous our accomplishments may seem to be, the attainment of supernatural powers should not be a source of self-importance. Even if we are blessed with the ability to perform incredible feats like walking on fire, placing our foot behind our head in yoga, or winning the gold in the Olympics, these feats should not define us or fuel our ego.

When we are attached to being praised or flattered, separation from self is impossible. To avoid suffering, remain diligent to earlier lessons. Stay grounded and detached (**vairāgyā**) regardless of successes, setbacks, or the admiration of others. By remaining in a state of equanimity, we nurture humility and stay focused on the joy that arises from a dedicated practice. True freedom comes only from letting go.

Sit comfortably with your back straight and your eyes closed. Take a few deep breaths, inhaling slowly and exhaling fully. Visualize yourself accomplishing a remarkable feat, achieving a long-held goal, or receiving recognition for your work. Notice any feelings of attachment that arise. Imagine yourself floating above the concepts of success and failure, detached from the need for external validation.

Picture the vast expanse of the sky, representing the boundless nature of your true self beyond the transient achievements of the world. As you breathe in, absorb the energy of humility and release any lingering attachments to accolades or accomplishments as you exhale. Feel a sense of lightness and inner freedom, recognizing that your worth extends far beyond the recognition or praise of others. Take a few more deep breaths and visualize yourself in a state of complete freedom, unattached to any external achievements. Nurture the essence of this inner liberation bringing equanimity and grace to your being.

3.53 to 3.56
Viveka jñāna
Divine Knowledge

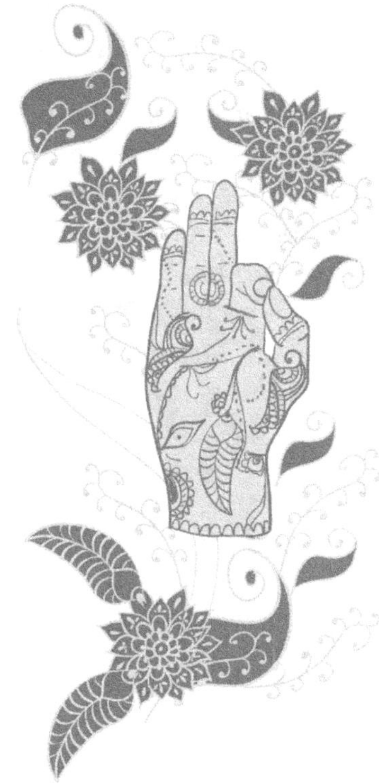

Discernment is the ability to see things for what they REALLY are and not for what you WANT them to be.

- Thich Nhat Hanh -

3.53

Kṣaṇa-tat-kramayoḥ **saṁyamad viveka-jam jñānaṁ.**

By practicing **saṁyama** on the continuous flow of moments (**ksana**), one attains profound insight (**jñāna**) born from discrimination (**vivekajam**).

Like the endless flow of a serene stream, as we remain witnesses to the infinite flow of moments, we weave this flowing spirit into our daily lives. Through the steady practice of *saṁyama* on this continuous flow, we gain access to the gift of **viveka**, supreme insight beyond our day-to-day knowledge.

Divine insight guides us to make wiser choices. We now understand the difference between the moment-by-moment (**kṣaṇa**), ever-changing nature of the material world—and the unchanging essence of *puruṣa* that resides beyond it. Like a meditation on a serene stream, there is much wisdom to be seen in the stillness of a single moment when we are awake in the Now.

In our present field of awareness, we no longer cling to fleeting and impermanent aspects of life, knowing that they are but ripples on the water's surface. Instead, through samyama on **kṣaṇa,** we find solace and wisdom in the changeless essence that exists beneath the ever-shifting surface of life's constant flux.

Practice Now in your meditative seat and observe the ceaseless flow of moments. Take notice of your ability to maintain focus undisturbed by external distractions or internal thoughts. Do not look back with your gaze. Do not look ahead. When challenging thoughts arise, acknowledge them, then let them go like leaves floating by on a stream. Remain steadfast in the present moment, and allow the current of awareness to carry you peacefully along the stream of life.

Enjoy this meditation *Leaves on a Stream* by Not Another Meditation. (*Scan QR code*)

3.54

Jāti-lakṣaṇa-deśair anyatā navacchedāt tulyayos tataḥ pratipattiḥ.

By discriminating between the characteristics (**jāti**), type (**lakṣaṇa**), and location (**deśa**), of things, the yogi gains the ability to recognize the difference between the ever-changing and the changeless.

Through divine insight (*viveka*) the yogi comprehends the impermanence of all things. Everything turns to dust eventually, just as clay, while taking various forms like pots, vases, and sculptures, ultimately returns to its original state. Understanding this greater meaning, we begin to recognize that life's abundance isn't measured by the accumulation of things, or by our accomplishments, but by the depth of our awareness and the connection to the changeless essence within.

As we detach from the material world, we find true freedom that arises from recognizing the eternal amidst the impermanent. Guided by our discernment, we are no longer attached to fleeting objects and discover richness in the abundance within. No longer grasping for life, we find contentment in the simple things and remember that we are *human beings, not human doings.*

Find a mindful seat in nature, maybe next to a flowing stream. Reflect on your desire to simplify life. Contemplate where you need to say 'no' instead of 'yes' to lighten your load. As you do, sense the freedom and lightness that simplicity brings. Feel the mind settling, releasing the need for constant mental chatter and busyness. Take this time to simply 'be' without the burden of 'doing.' In this quietude, notice that which is constant, like the steady flow of a stream, and that which is ever-changing. Feel the contentment and internal abundance that this stillness carries.

3.55

*Tārakam sarva-viṣayam sarvathā-viṣayam akramam
ceti viveka-jam jñānaṁ*

The transcendent (**tārakam**) knowledge born of higher discrimination, (**viveka-jam jñānaṁ**) is a great liberator. Insight includes the knowledge of all things in all moments.

From childhood, we naturally acquire knowledge. We learn the language of our culture, we study the intricacies of science and absorb the rituals of a particular religion. This knowledge is, of course, relevant in our daily lives, but it also holds us captive to the confines of the relative world.

When we connect with supreme insight born from discrimination, we flourish, living our highest potential. Under the influence of divine wisdom, **viveka-jñāna**, our tether to the material world and its patterns of thinking are undone.

Through yoga practice, we break free from our confines and open ourselves to the expansive vista of **tārakam**—transcendent knowledge. With the attainment of this *siddhi,* we move beyond the bounds of ordinary knowledge and embrace the infinite wisdom of the universe.

Chants to the goddess Saraswati invoke divine wisdom, seeking her guidance and blessings on the path of knowledge and enlightenment. Saraswati is revered as the embodiment of learning, wisdom, and the arts. She is seated on a lotus, symbolizing purity and transcendence. Saraswati holds the sacred scriptures, a veena (a traditional Indian string instrument), and a *mālā*, representing knowledge, creativity, and spirituality respectively. As the patroness of education and creativity, Saraswati is invoked by students, scholars, artists, and seekers alike, seeking her blessings to excel in their pursuits and attain inner wisdom.

Devotees chant the following Saraswati *bīja* mantra to invoke the wisdom of Saraswati:

Om Shreem Hreem Saraswatyai Namaha

In the divine presence of Saraswati, I offer my reverence and seek blessings for knowledge, wisdom, and creativity.

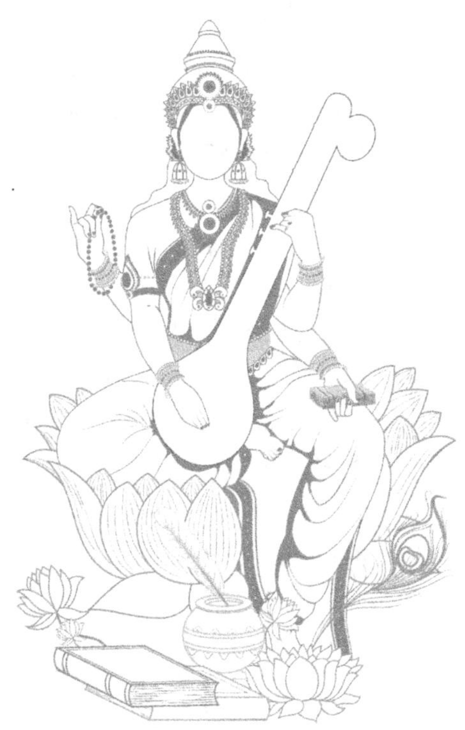

Awaken your seeds of wisdom with this guided meditation *The Seed Activation, Awakening Consciousness* by Niccolò Angeli of Kyrian and chant *The Saraswati Mahalo* by Daphne Tse. (*Scan QR code*)

3.56
Sattva puruṣayoḥ śuddhi sāmye kaivalyamiti.

When a tranquil mind (**sattva**) is equal in purity to the Self (**puruṣa**) then there is liberation–**kaivalya**.

The potential of the human mind is infinite. Its capacity unfolds through the ongoing process of perceiving and meditating on **puruṣa**.

By turning inward to meditate, we expand our awareness and experience the intricate workings of the natural world (*prakṛti*). We reach a state of **samādhi** in which the pure *sattvic* mind becomes one with the universal Self. No longer bound to the cycle of birth and death, true liberation from **prakṛti** is attained–the ultimate Freedom of **kaivalya**. It is here where we find a home in our True Self.

As you continue on your yogic journey, remember that you are capable of greatness beyond your imagination. Stay humbly committed to the practice, continuing to learn and grow, knowing your divinity within is waiting to be discovered. With Patanjali's practical guidance, you can attain **kaivalya** and experience the ultimate Freedom it offers.

So let's dive into the fourth and final chapter, **Kaivalya** Pāda.

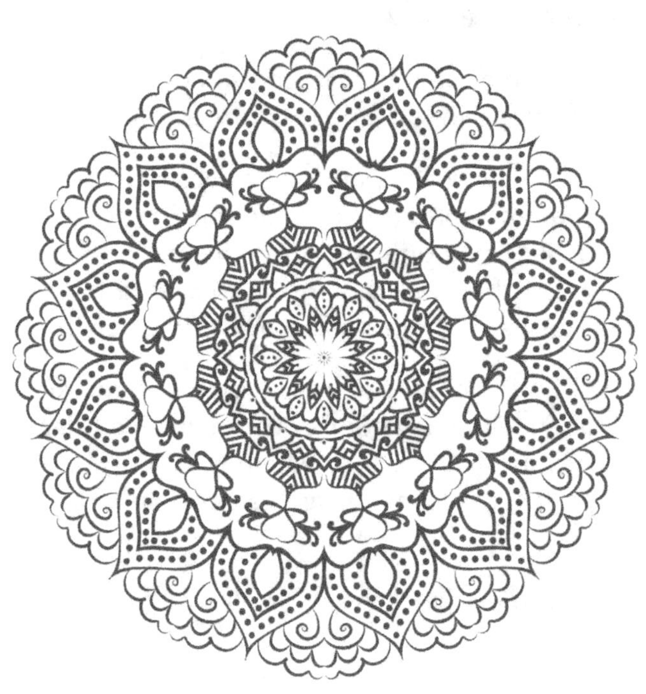

Chapter Four
Kaivalya Pāda
The Path to Freedom

Kaivalya is rooted in the word "isolation," *kevala*. It signifies our separation from the external world and our return to immersion with the pure essence of our being, our *puruṣa*. In *Pāda Four*, we encounter the unshakable, timeless Self. It is here that we will explore the transformative path that leads us closer to this state of Infinite Bliss. Let us continue together, embracing the wisdom of yoga and the infinite Freedom that awaits.

- On Evolution, Transformation and Reincarnation (4.1 to 4.12)
- Manifestations of Prakṛti (4.13 to 4.21)
- Draṣṭuḥ Svarūpe 'Vasthānam: At Rest in our True Nature (4.22 to 4.28)
- Dharmameghḥ Samādhi: Cloud of Virtues (4.29 to 4.32)
- Kaivalya: Liberation (4.33 to 4.34)

4.1 to 4.12
On Evolution, Transformation, and Reincarnation

Every day, think as you wake up, today, I am fortunate to be alive,
I have a precious human life, I am not going to waste it. I am going
to use all my energies to develop myself, to expand my heart out to
others; to achieve enlightenment for the benefit of all beings.

- Dalai Lama -

4.1
Janmauṣadhi mantra tapḥ samādhijāḥ siddhayḥ.

Siddhis can arise from birth, herbs, **mantra** repetition, **tapas** and **samādhi**.

From Pāda Three, we learned about the extraordinary capacity of our minds with the *siddhis* of yoga. As we move into the inner world of *kaivalya*, Patanjali begins by explaining that mystical gifts can arise from many sources, including:

- birth (**janma**)
- elixirs (**oṣadhi**)
- incantation (**mantra**)
- self-discipline (**tapas**)
- enlightenment (**samādhi**)

This distinction reminds us that to successfully walk the Raja Yoga path, we must keep the aim of yoga in the forefront of our minds. Our goal as a practitioner is not to become distracted by the pursuit of mystical powers, but to end our suffering by removing the veil of ignorance and connecting with supreme insight. Though there are many ways to access gifts, the path to **samādhi** is one.

As real-life inspiration, we can look to the life of Ram Das, an influential spiritual philosopher. Initially, a Harvard professor who experimented with psychedelic drugs during the 1960s, Ram Das underwent an internal shift when he encountered his spiritual teacher, Neem Karoli Baba, during a visit to India. Inspired, Ram Das embarked on a journey of self-discovery separate from external substances, where he learned that true wisdom comes from within. He eventually became a revered spiritual teacher himself.

Watch the documentary *Ram Das, Going Home*. Like Ram Das, through introspection and conscious living, we too can find Freedom. (*Scan QR code*)

4.2

Jātyantarapariṇāmḥ prakṛtyāpūrāt

Transformation (**pariṇāma**) through rebirth (**jātya**) is determined by one's *saṁskāras*.

Each misstep is an opportunity to learn through experience. In our errors, we discover ways to avoid negative actions in the present, cultivate good *karma*, and pave the way for a more positive tomorrow. In our capacity to face our mistakes and our *saṁskāras*, we reshape our understanding of the past and influence the decisions of our future selves.

Think of it like the evolution of a species over the generations—just as organisms adapt and evolve over time to better suit their environments, we, through our conscious actions and intentions, direct the ongoing process of the spiritual evolution of our *citta*. Every choice we make and every action we take affects our progress of self-unfoldment in this lifetime and in the next.

The practice of yoga offers us the means to mold our future selves through conscious awareness. Recall *sutra* 2.33 and the practice of **pratipakṣa bhāvanam**, cultivation of opposites, an exercise that turns negative thoughts into positive ones. At any point in our journey, we can turn things around. We can inspire **pariṇāma** by engaging in yogic practices that help us reexamine our past scars, shift perspective, and move forward. By taking the steps that lead to transformation, we become the directors of our own evolution, ultimately liberating ourselves from the cycle of rebirth.

So let us do good in this life, enriching our spirits, transforming our hearts, and leading to even more enlightened **pariṇāma** in the next.

4.3

Nimittam aprayojakam prakṛtīnām varaṇabhedastu taṭh kṣetrikavat.

Transformation arises by changing our inner nature, just like the farmer removes obstacles in the way of his irrigation system.

As we eliminate obstacles, our true essence unfolds. Recall the five *kleśas* (*Sūtra 2.3*): *avidyā* (unawareness), *asmitā* (ego), *rāga* (attachment), *dveṣa* (aversion), and *abhiniveśāḥ* (clinging to fear). The *kleśas* are like weeds in the field of our consciousness. By recognizing these deterrents, we transform ourselves from within and move closer to the ultimate goal of *kaivalya*.

Come back to your lily pad and become the radiant lotus flower. Close your eyes and feel the depth of murkiness and muck below your true Self.

Visualize the mud beneath you as the challenges, negative thoughts and limiting beliefs that perhaps cloud your mind. Breathe in deeply and imagine the lotus roots growing from the core of your being, nurturing your inner beauty amidst the murky waters. Feel the strong roots of your resilience and inner strength, even in the darkness, and connect with your ability to push through obstacles.

Now, focus on your lotus petals, see them opening one by one to reveal your authentic inner radiance. As each petal unfurls, imagine any layers of self-doubt and negativity falling away. As you sit, serene in the murk, see how you rise above challenges, magnificent and whole. You are the lotus, and your true Self remains pure and luminous.

Remember that transformation is a journey that requires patience, perseverance, and a willingness to sit with our inner demons. Become the radiant lotus flower with this practice by the Floating Yoga School. (*Scan QR code*)

4.4

Nirmāṇacittānyasmitāmātrāt.

Transformation may be limited if the yogi's ego (**asmitā**) gets in the way of the free mind.

The ego represents the part of our mind that seeks validation, recognition, and a sense of identity through external sources. **Asmitā** (Sūtra 2.5) is our "I-Ness" that attaches itself to the roles we play, defining us by them and creating a sense of separateness and individuality.

In our day-to-day lives, we take on roles such as mother, father, friend or professional. These labels are, of course, the reality of our existence, but by identifying solely with the ego and the roles it assumes, we limit our potential for growth and expansion. While our function and purpose in society have meaning, transformation and true liberation occur only when we recognize the transitory nature of these roles, and detach our sense of self-worth from them.

By disentangling ourselves from the ego's identification with roles, we cultivate inner joy and authenticity. This does not mean negating or abandoning our responsibilities, but rather approaching them from a place of inner spaciousness and non-attachment. We can engage in our responsibilities wholeheartedly while understanding that they are temporary expressions of our being, not the entirety of who we are.

Through self-inquiry, meditation, and self-reflection, we begin to discern between the ego's need for validation and that which is authentic and True. With this shift comes greater joy and creativity in all that we are and all that we aspire to be.

Join Anand Ji in releasing the ego with *Effortless Presence* by Sattva Connect. (*Scan QR code*)

4.5
*Pravṛttibhede prayojakam **citta**eka**manekeṣām.***

The one (**eka**) Self is the director of all the many states of the mind (***citta***).

Just as a skilled conductor leads an orchestra, our inner Self holds the baton, guiding and harmonizing the cacophony of thoughts, emotions, and desires into a beautiful and coherent melody. This one unified Self, the core essence of our being, gracefully governs the fluctuations or *vṛittis* of the mind.

Recall a challenging situation that triggered feelings of frustration or anger. If you reacted impulsively, give yourself grace as you continually expand through the process of self-realization. As we delve deeper into the process, we become aware of the underlying source beneath the layers of our emotions. Instead of burning in the heat of past anger, yoga teaches us to approach the situation with discernment, and respond thoughtfully rather than react impulsively.

Through yoga, we become continual *Witnesses* of the world around us. When we reconnect with the Self and allow it to be our guiding force, we become less reactive and learn to self-direct the orchestra of our mind towards greater harmony and equanimity. Ultimately, we emerge as Witnesses of *all* our interactions.

By practicing *svādyāya* and reading more about mindfulness and meditation, such as *The Power of Now* by Eckhart Tolle or *Mindfulness in Plain English* by Bhante Gunaratana, we can deepen our understanding of this *sūtra*. (*Scan QR code*)

4.6

*Tatra **dhyānajam** anāśayaṁ.*

From these [many states of the mind], the one born of meditation is without the storehouse of *karma*.

The more we engage in meditation, the more we grow our storehouse (*karmāsayo*) of positive impressions. When our daily routine reflects this meditative state (**dhyāna**), a unique form of awareness emerges called **dhyānajam**. This meditative form of knowledge is devoid of any lingering imprints or biases from past experiences or conditioning.

As the whirlwind of the *vṛttis* calms, there is a quieting of ignorance (*avidyā*). Where once we were entangled in the stories and demands of the ego, through yoga we become indifferent Witnesses to the interactions around us. What once was perceived as stressful and overwhelming, we now begin to view with a sense of equanimity.

Spend a day increasing your time in meditation, as though every moment were a meditation. As you go about your daily activities, make a conscious effort to anchor your awareness in the present moment. Every time your mind begins to wander or get lost in thoughts of the past or future, bring yourself back to the Now and repeat to yourself:

"I am awake with loving kindness in the present moment."

Allow the words to resonate within you. Feel their significance and depth as they become a gentle, yet powerful reminder to connect with this moment. Notice the sensations in your body, the sounds around you, and the details of your surroundings. Experience the richness of the Now as it fills your being.

Continue this mindful state with *Be The Witness* by The Mindful Movement and Becoming the Witness with YoEddie. (*Scan QR code*)

4.7

Karmāśuklākṛṣṇam yoginastrividhamitareṣām.

For the yogi, **karma** is neither white (good-*śuklā*) nor black (bad *ākṛṣṇa*), for others it is three-fold.

Most people find life to be pleasurable, painful or a mixture of both pleasure and pain. For the yogi, these distinctions dissolve.

The experiences of life now transcend the classification of positive or negative. The yogi is no longer subject to the fluctuations and uncertainties of life's ups and downs. As duality ceases to exist, everything becomes a translucent reflection of the Self.

The path to becoming less reactive and more responsive is a gradual process that unfolds through dedicated practice. Previously entangled in cycles of judgment and personal perceptions, the yogic path cultivates discernment, understanding, and acceptance. Deepening awareness liberates us to witness life unfolding without the constraints of preconceived notions.

Through this shift, we open ourselves to the vast spectrum of experiences, recognizing each moment as an opportunity for growth and self-awareness. This transformation does not merely occur through intellectual understanding but rather through the awakening of our energetic centers and the change in the molecular structure of our brains, nurtured by consistent practice.

Challenge yourself to spend an entire day or even a week without labeling anything as "good" or "bad"—even your favorite dessert. Simply observe your experiences without judgment, witnessing life as it unfolds without trying to control the flow of moments. Notice the changes within you as you practice non-judgmental awareness, feeling a sense of equanimity and gratitude towards all experiences, whether positive or negative.

4.8

Tatastadvipākānuguṇānāmevābhivyaktirvāsanānām

Of these actions follows the manifestation of only those **vāsanās** (subliminal traits) for which there are favorable conditions for producing their fruits.

Deep within our consciousness lie imprints from past experiences that give rise to habitual patterns or enduring personality traits (**vāsanās**). Our actions, thoughts, and reactions shape our karma, and the seeds of potential blossom when the circumstances around us nurture the positive karma waiting to manifest.

The scenarios of our lives bear great significance in producing positive karma. We can be certain that healthy habits develop only under healthy circumstances and the right opportunities. Through our work with the *yāmas* and *niyamas*, we have already seen how our surroundings and the company we keep play a crucial role in the journey towards self-realization.

Our environment molds and guides our karma, either supporting or hindering our spiritual progress. For instance, consider a tendency towards pessimism. It would be challenging to avoid karma resulting from this mindset in an environment that fosters negativity and cynicism. Whereas an environment that promotes positivity and optimism may be the perfect nurturing soil for this person to thrive.

Take note of your environment and your surroundings. Notice which books are on your shelf, What is hanging on your walls? What music do you listen to? What are you feeding your mind with online? Are your surroundings peaceful promoting a healthy body and mind? Reflect on your relationships. How do they support or hinder your growth? How can you seek like-minded individuals and release detrimental relationships?

4.9

Jāti deśa kāla vyavahitānām apyānantaryam smṛti saṁskārayorekarūpatvāt.

Despite differences in our birth (**jāti**), place (**deśa**), and time (**kāla**), there is a continuous connection of our memories (**smṛti**) and thoughts (**saṁskāra**) making our consciousness an unbroken flow.

All of who we are and what we experience, all of what we were and will become work together to bring us to Self-Realization.

Our memories and impressions are an integral part of our journey. According to the teachings, the experiences and impressions we accumulate in our lives continue to shape and guide us throughout our subsequent incarnations.

This truth may inspire us to explore practices such as hypnosis and shamanic energy healing of past life trauma. Brian Weiss in his book *Many Lives, Many Masters* shares stories of patients undergoing past-life regression, uncovering deep-seated fears and patterns originating from previous lifetimes. By addressing these impressions, we pave the way for healing across time and space, allowing for healing in our present life. By embracing these ancient teachings and modern modalities, wisdom flows through the ages, guiding us towards the ultimate realization of our true Nature.

Imagine yourself as a fetus in the sacred space of the womb. Sense the loving and nurturing energy that surrounds you. Inhale deeply absorbing the essence of this space. Sense the connection to the memories and impressions from your past lives. Envision a radiant golden thread extending from your current self to the core of your being in previous lifetimes. Picture the people and events along this golden thread, and observe the emotions it stirs within you. With each breath, allow this golden thread to illuminate, carrying with it the wisdom, lessons, and strengths gained from your past experiences. Sense the interweaving of lifetimes, and the interconnectedness of your existence. Acknowledge the growth and transformation that transcends time.

4.10

Tāsāmanāditvam cāśiṣo nityatvāt.

Human desire is eternal and consequently so are *vāsanās* (personality traits).

Consider the desires that have accompanied your life. The longing for love, the pursuit of knowledge, the ambition to succeed—these desires don't appear out of nowhere. They are born from your *vāsanās*, which, as the *sūtra* reminds us, are without beginning or end. Our *vāsanās*, our deep-rooted personality traits, are the imprints left by our eternal desires on our psyche. These inclinations and tendencies influence our thoughts, actions and reactions.

Recognizing the eternal nature of *vāsanās* allows us to approach our desires with greater understanding and self-compassion. We can acknowledge that though our desires are not easily extinguished or suppressed, we can work with them, transforming them into positive forces that guide us towards our fullest potential and spiritual evolution.

Close your eyes and take a few breaths. Begin to internally describe your personality traits and desires, first beginning with those that are positive. Say to yourself—I am compassionate, I am funny, I desire peace for all humanity etc. Notice how it feels in your body as you celebrate these positive traits. Now dig deeper and ask yourself what are your negative personality traits and desires such as I am jealous, I am powered by money, I crave attention. Now let all that go and just repeat I am, I am, I am… so'ham, so'ham, so'ham…

You are your true Spirit—that is all. Continue to find peace in this mantra by coming back to it over and over again.

Join Mooji in *Discovering Freedom*. (*Scan QR code*)

4.11

Hetu phalāśrayālambanaiḥ saṃgṛhītatvādeṣāmabhāve tadabhāvḥ.

When the building blocks of *vāsanās*—cause, motive, the *karmasayo*, and external stimulation—are no longer present, the *vāsanās* naturally fade away.

Without our conscious awareness, we become blind to the influence our *vāsanās* exert on our thoughts, emotions, and behaviors. This can create a vicious cycle of repetitive, ingrained patterns that reinforce our self-harming tendencies. Through disciplined meditation, we become aware of and remove *vāsanās* that are harmful to our wellbeing. We break the chain of cause and effect, freeing ourselves from our conditioned patterns of behavior.

Consider the tendency to carry excessive worry or anxiety. This unease tightly grips our minds, and leads to tension in our thoughts and fear in our actions. Through each *conscious breath*, we create something new. By bringing ourselves back over and over again to our mats for mantra, movement and meditation a shift within occurs. There is a gradual awakening inside of us, and fear gives way to a heartfelt sense of calm and resilience.

Try this *prāṇāyāma* practice called "transformational breath" for stress and anxiety.

Find a comfortable position. Close your eyes and place your hands on your belly. Open the mouth wide, and take a full and complete inhale, and then a full and complete exhale. Make sure you can hear yourself breathing. Continue for 50 breaths, keeping the mouth gently open wide. Gradually increase the time and notice the sweet release from worry.

Here is a powerful healing breathwork session called *Rise of the Phoenix*, by *Dakota Earth Cloud Walker*, Insight Timer. (*Scan QR code*)

4.12

*Atītānāgatam **svarūpa**to'styadhvabhedāddharmāṇām.*

Both the past and the future are inherent in one's own Nature (**svarūpa**).

Our very existence is intertwined with the natural cycle of birth, life, death, and rebirth. Just as a beautiful flower exists within a seed, or a wilted plant has the potential to grow anew, this ancient wisdom invites us to embrace the rhythmic dance of life—the melodious interplay of past, present, and future that is an inseparable part of our being.

This wisdom reminds us that just as the past and the future are embedded in our very nature, so too is our ability to transcend our struggles and challenges. By embracing the present moment and learning to trust in the flow of the universe, *kṣaṇa* by *kṣaṇa*, little by little, we can find the strength to face and overcome obstacles with grace and resilience.

Find a mindful seat, sit tall and center yourself. Reflect on a situation in your life that you've been resisting or struggling against. It could be a difficult relationship, a challenging work project, or a health issue. Now, close your eyes and take a deep breath. Repeat the following mantra to yourself:

"I am a part of the natural cycle of life. I trust in the flow of the universe and let go of resistance. I embrace the present moment and allow life to unfold."

Take a few more deep breaths and visualize yourself flowing with the natural cycle of life. See yourself letting go of resistance and embracing the present moment with ease and grace. Like Shiva dancing in the cosmos, allow Nature to do her work and experience the beauty inherent in the flow of the universe.

4.13 to 4.21
Manifestations of Prakṛti

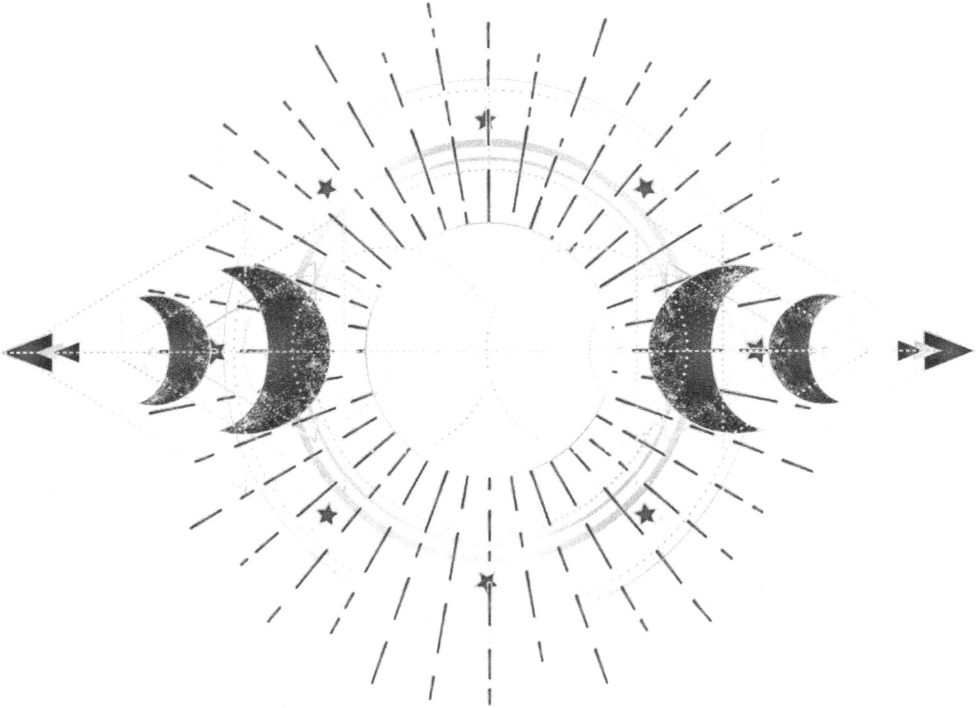

Tap into your subconscious, and you master yourself.
Tap into the quantum, and you master your life.

- Brooke Nally -

4.13

Te vyaktasūkṣmāḥ guṇātmānḥ.

All of existence, whether manifest or subtle (**sūkṣmā**), are expressions of the three **guṇā.**

These **guṇas**, *rajas, tamas, and sattva,* as explained in previous *sūtras* (1.16, 2.18, and 2.19), are the building blocks of the universe. Whether expressing actualized energy or potential energy, every aspect of existence is characterized by the interplay of the **guṇas**.

These interacting forces of energy are seen in all manifestations of existence. They reveal themselves in the hustle and bustle of a city or conversely in the tranquil slumber of a sleeping baby. *Rajas* shows itself in a heated argument or in the passion of an artist fully immersed in the creative process. *Tamas* is revealed in a neglected space or a person consumed by heaviness. We experience *sattva* during a meditative state of mind when radiating inner peace.

These forces also exist outside the individual, and can be witnessed in the aura of a tranquil forest, the stillness and *sattva* of a calm ocean or the *rajas* of a stormy day. The ancient teachings of yoga and Samkhya philosophy remind us that, even beyond the human world, everything in the universe is part of the same interconnected, fundamental energy, whether those forces manifest or remain unmanifested karmically.

*Take a few moments to reflect on your current state of mind and emotions. Notice any feelings of restlessness, lethargy, or imbalance. Now, close your eyes and take a deep breath. As you exhale, release any tension or negativity from your body and mind. Next, visualize the three **guṇas** as three colored lights: green for rajas, red for tamas, and white for sattva. See these lights swirling around you, intermingling and affecting your energy. Notice which **guṇa** feels dominant in your energy field. Is it rajas, tamas, or sattva? Without judgment, simply observe and acknowledge the condition of your current state.*

4.14

Pariṇāmaikatvādvastutattvam

The reality of an object is due to the transformations (**pariṇāma**) of the three *guṇas*.

When we look at form on a molecular level, the same building blocks are found in the human, the monkey, the bird and all aspects of nature. The remarkable interplay of atoms stands as an amazing expression of scientific marvel in the unique ways molecules come together to shape the grand diversity witnessed in our natural world. This perpetual biological and metaphysical transformation unfolds seamlessly, guided by the dynamic forces of *rajas*, *tamas*, and *sattva*.

Even amidst this extraordinary diversity, the wisdom of the yoga *sūtras* reminds us that beneath all variations lies the same fundamental unity. Transcending the expressions of the *guṇas* is the Seer or *draṣṭā* (sūtra 2.20), the pure consciousness that connects everything in the universe. It is the singular essence that binds all elements in the manifest and unmanifest worlds.

Patanjali teaches that all of Nature (*prakṛti*) exists for the purposes of the Seer (*sūtra* 2.21). As we grasp the Oneness of all existence, even in the face of grand diversity, true Freedom reveals itself.

Repeat the following mantra to yourself:

"I honor the diversity and uniqueness of all beings and everything in the natural world. I recognize that although we come from the same source, we express ourselves in different and beautiful ways. I embrace the Oneness that unites us all."

Join Megan Shirey with *Earthly Diversity* to accompany this *sūtra*.
(*Scan QR code*)

4.15

*Vastusāmye **citta** bhedāt tayorvibhaktḥ panthāḥ.*

Because all minds (**citta**) are different, the same object may be perceived differently.

On the surface, one may see the human, the monkey, or the bird as being different from each other. As we reach deeper into the depths of our subconscious, a shift in our perspective occurs. The human, monkey and bird are now understood as composed of the same fundamental material. The yogi, finely attuned to the subtleties of existence, begins to perceive all facets of life from diverse angles and perspectives.

When our mind is clear and balanced, it can better perceive the subtle manifestations of the *guṇas*. In other words, we can better see the interplay of *rajas*, *tamas*, and *sattva*, and how their forces affect our experiences. For example, a storm from a purely *rajasic* perspective may appear chaotic and destructive. From a *tamasic* viewpoint, one might quietly hide from the storm. In a *sattvic* state, however, one might see the grand beauty in the natural forces of nature.

Now the Seer (*draṣṭā*) begins to observe the seen (*dṛśyam*) from a whole different view.

Through this panoramic vision, the yogi aligns with a profound sense of Oneness that transcends the limitations of mere surface-level perception. When the mind is in a state of equanimity it can perceive an object as it truly is without being clouded by personal biases or tendencies.

4.16

*Na ca**ika citta** tantram vastu tad a**pramāṇa**kam tadā kim syāt*

An object's existence does not depend on one (**eka**) single mind (**citta**).

An enlightened yogi may no longer perceive a tree as a tree but may now perceive it from a subatomic level. So if the tree disappears for an enlightened yogi it does not mean that it disappears for another. At the subtlest level, the tree doesn't exist, but on the surface level it will continue to exist, illustrating the different levels of reality and perception.

Gifted with the understanding of the union between the Seer and the seen (*sūtra* 2.23), we recognize that the nature of reality is separate from our individual lens. Instead of approaching our universe from one perspective, we begin to define our reality through the eyes of the collective consciousness. In this deeper connection with our subtle body and the larger universe, the subtleties underlying the reality of our existence are revealed.

Sages, rishis, and shamanic teachers help guide us to sense the interconnectedness of all things. When we move deeper into the subconscious mind, our perception changes. Now we look at our reality in a completely different way, even finding life in inanimate objects. By recognizing that our perception of our material world is shaped by our minds, rather than objective truth, we break down the barriers that connect and separate us from each other, and from the deeper layers of existence.

Find a quiet space and hold a meaningful object in your hands. It could be a special stone, small statue or pottery. Close your eyes and sense the object. How does the weight of the object make you feel? What emotions arise as you sense its texture? Can you sense the energy radiating from it? What significance and connection does this object hold for you? What memories or emotions does it evoke? Express gratitude for the object and any guidance it may provide. Open your eyes, carrying the object's energy into the present moment.

Expand your awareness by taking this shamanic journey. (*Scan QR code*)

4.17

*Taduparāgāpekṣitvāc**citta**sya vastu jñātājñātaṁ.*

Recognition and awareness of something or an object happens only when the mind (**citta**) can perceive it.

Even though human beings are unable to perceive certain phenomena, such as the true color of the sky or certain sound waves outside our hearing range, the practice of yoga carries the possibility of developing *siddhis* that awaken new dimensions of perception. Once we evolve these deeper levels of awareness through meditation, our *citta* can see that which was once beyond its grasp.

Before we began our practice, our perception was limited, blinded by our strong connection to the relative world. Now, having removed *avidya*, we access higher states of consciousness that open us up to the infinite. With this awakening, we embrace the richness of life, cherishing the fullness of every moment.

Find a quiet and comfortable space. Close your eyes and take a few deep breaths, allowing yourself to enter a state of centered focus. Now, bring to mind something that you know exists but cannot perceive through your five senses. It could be a sound, an aroma, a color beyond your sensory range, or perhaps the ability of an animal to communicate feelings. Visualize this object or phenomenon in the mind's eye, and attempt to connect with it on an intuitive level.

Notice any sensations, emotions, or insights that arise as you direct your attention towards this object or sensation. After taking a few more deep breaths, slowly open your eyes, carrying this expanded awareness with you throughout your day.

Continue the practice with this hypnotherapy session called *Let Go, Beyond the Five Senses.* (*Scan QR code*)

4.18

Sadā jñātāścittavṛttayastatprabhoḥ **puruṣasyāpariṇāmitvāt**.

On the other hand **puruṣa** will always perceive a change in the mind-stuff (**cittavṛtti**) at the subtlest level.

While *prakṛti* undergoes constant transformation in various forms, including those forms which we cannot see, **puruṣa** remains changeless and eternal.

Prakṛti encompasses the entire realm of manifested existence, including our physical bodies, thoughts, emotions, and the external world. It is subject to constant flux and change, taking on different forms and expressions through the *guṇas*.

In contrast, **puruṣa** represents the unchanging, eternal essence of consciousness. It is that which is not thinking or processing, but simply *Witnessing* it all. It is the supreme Self beyond the transient nature of the material world. It is unlimited awareness even on the subtlest level, and that which observes the ever-changing *vṛittis* of the mind, yet remains untouched by them.

Ask yourself again, Who am I?

Am I my thoughts? Am I my thinking mind? Am I my suffering? Am I my joy? My sorrow? Am I the color of my skin? Am I my desires? Am I my profession? Am I my goals? Am I my sexual affiliation?

When we remove all these labels what is left?

Continue to explore that which lies beyond the transient nature of thoughts and perceptions, with this practice by Mooji, *Remain As You Are*. (*Scan QR code*)

4.19

Na tat svābāsam dṛśyatvāt.

The mind (*citta*) is not self-luminous or *puruṣa* because it has the ability to perceive things as good or bad.

Unlike *puruṣa*, the mind is not inherently enlightened because it possesses the capacity to discern and judge things as favorable or unfavorable, good or bad. The mind's ability to perceive duality and make value judgments indicates its dependence on external factors and reflects its limited nature.

While *puruṣa* remains ever-present within us, the *citta* will become entangled in negative thinking or distractions of the material world. By understanding that we are *puruṣa*, we regain our grounding and connect within our state of perennial Bliss. As promised in Sūtra 1.16, when you know your True Spirit (**puruṣa**), then you can completely detach from energies (*guṇas*) detrimental to your journey.

*Take a moment to sit in a quiet and comfortable space. Close your eyes and bring your attention inward. Recognize that the essence of who you truly are is **puruṣa**–the unchanging consciousness that exists beyond the fluctuations of the mind.*

Internally repeat the mantra,

"I am not my physical body, I am not my thinking mind."

Allow this affirmation to permeate your being as a reminder that your true identity transcends the limitations of the physical body and the transient nature of thoughts.

Continue this practice with *I Am Not My Body, I Am Not My Mind* (Sadhguru) by Brian Scott. (*Scan QR code*)

4.20

Ekasamaye cobhayānavadhāraṇaṁ

It is impossible for the mind to perceive the subject (*puruṣa*) and object (*prakṛti*) at the same time.

4.21

*Cittāntara dṛśye **buddhi**buddheratiprasaṅgḥ **smṛtisaṁkara**śca*

It is absurd that the mind (**cittā**) could observe the mind. This would imply the infinite deterioration of intelligence and confuse the memory.

It is impossible for the mind to observe the mind. We can only remain present and aware. Therefore, there must be something else observing the mind that is changeless.

Subtler than all the evolutes of *prakṛti*, including **buddhi** (higher awakening), **smṛti** (memory), and **ahaṁkara** (the ego), is the unchanging *puruṣa*. The *puruṣa* remains ever constant.

This is seemingly impossible to understand, but we can distinguish it in practice. By becoming aware of the unchanging observer, we detach ourselves from the ceaseless activity of the mind, ultimately experiencing the peace and clarity of the unchanging Self.

Join Mooji in this practice titled *The Power of Observing*. (*Scan QR code*)

4.22 to 4.28
Draṣṭuḥ Svarūpe Vasthānam
At Rest in Our True Nature

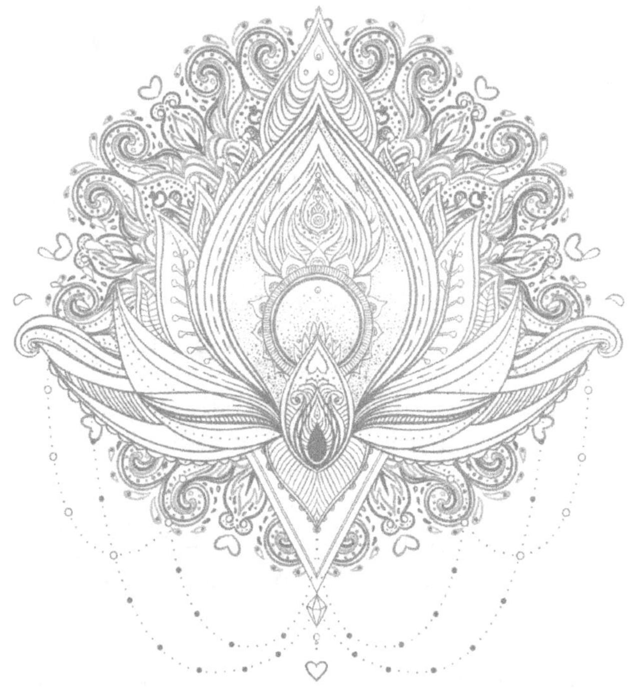

Your true nature is that of infinite spirit.
The feeling of limitation is the work of the mind.
- Ramana Maharshi -

4.22

*Citerapratisaṁkramāyāstadākārāpattau sva**buddhi**saṁvedanam.*

When the unchanging consciousness of the *puruṣa* reflects on the *citta*, the functioning of higher cognition (**buddhi**) becomes possible.

Buddhi is the part of our consciousness that embodies discernment and higher intelligence. Similar to the ever-present radiance of the full moon, or *chandra*, when *puruṣa* reflects upon the *citta*, **buddhi** emanates from our entire being.

Like the full moon, after which remains whole even when obscured by shadows during certain phases, with the awakening of **buddhi** we are reminded that we too are always "full" (*purna*), even in times of darkness. When we remain for extended periods in this awakened state, the light of cosmic consciousness unfolds. **Buddhi** kindles in us an understanding of our inherent divinity—the realization of being an eternal, unchanging spirit. Radiating like the *purna* of *chandra* and bathing in the light of our inner brilliance, we experience the fullness and the entirety of who we truly are.

Sit in stillness and imagine the full moon, its reflection dancing upon the waves of a serene ocean at dusk. Notice the reflection of the moon upon the water, the ripples sometimes causing a turbulent reflection. Notice, despite the ripples, the moon remains full and whole in the sky. This "purna" is always present within you. Feel the radiant light enveloping you, infusing every cell and thought with clarity and wisdom. In this expanded awareness, remember you are always "full."

Invoke the brilliance and peace of the full moon with the *chandra bija* mantra:

Om Shram Shreem Shroum Sah Chandramasé Namah

Om, I invoke the energy of the moon, reminding me of my inner shanti and fullness

Continue to awaken *purna* with this *Full Moon Meditation*, by the Yoga Institute. (*Scan QR code*)

4.23

Draṣṭṛ dṛśyoparaktam cittam sarvārtham.

When the pure mind or *buddhi* is colored by both the seen (**dṛśya**) and the Seer (**draṣṭṛ**), awareness becomes all-knowing (**sarvā**).

With the purity of *buddhi*, the mind now reflects the world without distortion. Where once the mind was colored only by a 3-dimensional limited reality, with only glimpses of the Seen, now it exists in beautiful harmony with the expansive and infinite shades of life. Like the pure reflection of the moon upon a still serene ocean, the awakened mind—the Seer (**draṣṭṛ**—pure awareness) and the seen (**dṛśya**- the material world) shine as One.

As we begin to observe the world through a broader lens, the mind becomes a luminous medium through which the vastness of existence becomes comprehensible. In this clarified state, ripples upon the wave of the ocean do not disturb the awareness of the yogi, whose peace shines even amidst adversity. When we find ourselves whole and complete—no longer in the shadows, like the radiant *"purna"* of the full moon—the mind expands into a boundless expanse of all-knowing.

In this state, the yogi is very close to reaching *kaivalya,* but if practice is not consistent, the yogi will fall back once again.

Continue your *steady* practice. Continue the involution of your highest Self.

Witness the expansiveness of *buddhi* with this meditation *Trust in Divine Wisdom.* (*Scan QR code*)

4.24

Tad asaṁkhyeyavāsanābhiścittamapi parārtham saṁhatyakāritvāt.

Although the mind (**citta**) fluctuates due to personality traits (**vāsanā**) and countless desires, the **citta** works in association with *puruṣa*.

The mind exists either to provide experience or liberation. This is where we have a choice. The mind can persist on auto-pilot, guided by **vāsanās** pulling the mind towards objects, senses, and desires, or, alternatively, it can seek spiritual solace through self-unfoldment.

Through practice, the mind is no longer subservient to *prakṛti* and becomes an agent of *puruṣa*. By continually exercising the muscle of our mind, not only do negative **vāsanās** lose their grip, but the incredible transformations that we learned in Pada 3 fully emerge. The yogi becomes a powerful *siddha*, strong, stable and *complete*.

Regardless of the time invested in practice, we cannot become complacent. The yogi must continue with strict discipline, otherwise, the *vrittis*, the *kleśas*, and *vāsanās* will continue to persist. Consistent, steady practice is the key to transformation—*Master the mind, and you master your life.*

Keep practicing. Here are three more practices according to level. (*Scan QR code*)

Beginner: *Yoga for Complete Beginners*, Yoga with Adriene
Intermediate: *Breathing into Blissful Being*, Boho Beautiful
Advanced: *Best Kundalini Class to Balance all Chakras*, Akhanda Yoga Institute with Dr. Yogrishi Vishvketu

4.25

Viśeṣadarśina ātmabhāva bhāvanā vinivṛttiḥ.

When the yogi can distinguish (**viśeṣa**) between the **ātma** and the mind, self-consciousness ceases.

When we dive deep into the depths of our consciousness, we meet the timeless *ātma*, the spark of *puruṣa* and the part of ourselves untouched by the fleeting aspects of the *citta*. Through this encounter with our true spirit, we move towards *kaivalya*.

Find a quiet and comfortable space for self-reflection. Close your eyes and bring your attention inward. Come back to the question, "Who am I?"

If everything could be removed from your mind, every memory, thought, feeling, dream, attachment so that you are totally empty what do you observe?

Notice the thoughts and sensations that arise without judgment or attachment. Observe that these mental and physical experiences come and go, while there is a deeper sense of presence and awareness that remains constant. Feel your thoughts and emotions melting away as you recognize that they are not the true essence of your being. You are the constant and complete observer of the mind's fluctuations. You are the eternal **ātma** *free from the ever-changing mind. You are complete as you are…*

Continue focusing on Divine Consciousness with Eckhart Tolle's meditation, *You Are the Consciousness of the Universe*. (*Scan QR code*)

4.26

*Tadā hi **viveka**nimnam **kaivalya** prāgbhāram **cittam***

Then the mind with clearer discernment (**viveka**) moves towards Absoluteness (**kaivalya**).

When we recognize that we are the *ātman* and not all the manifestations of our three-dimensional world, then we can move towards Absoluteness. Our ego-driven life is full of repetitive cycles and suffering, but through discernment and self-awareness (**viveka**), we break free from these patterns and move towards a life of greater meaning and value.

Anand Ji, owner of Sattva Yoga School in Rishikesh, India, sums up this *sutra* perfectly:

"Only when one sees one's own folly clearly can one see the possibility of liberation. That's when one gets interested. The individual gets interested in liberation, in kaivalya... our ego life is a life of vāsanās and it has no meaning. You are running around, you feel bad, you feel good, you like someone, you don't like someone, you try to get a job, you don't get a job, today you feel great, the day after tomorrow you feel awful, It's the same and it's pointless. This is the endless cycle."[5]

True liberation arises when one sees their own folly clearly. An awakened consciousness transcends the superficial fluctuations of emotions and pursuits, ultimately leading to the embrace of the Absolute.

Move towards Absoluteness with this practice with Anand Ji. (*Scan QR code*)

4.27

*Tacchidreṣu **pratyayāntarāṇi samskā**rebhyḥ*

With the veils of **samskāras** removed, new mental impressions (**pratyayā**) may at times arise.

During meditation, the yogi may suddenly become aware of an arising thought (**pratyayā**), which has surfaced from the subconscious mind. These thoughts may unearth deeply rooted emotional pain and trigger difficult feelings, but with *viveka* the *citta* gains clarity that enables the yogi to detach from these thoughts with non-judgmental awareness.

The yogi's journey involves an ongoing cycle of progress, setbacks, progress, setbacks. As more **samskāras** are lifted, this process becomes progressively more manageable. The *citta* gradually releases its grip, and the mind becomes free like the vastness of the clear blue sky.

Detaching oneself from deeply ingrained patterns requires patience, persistence, and a willingness to confront and transcend one's conditioning. Each step forward, however difficult, brings the yogi closer to a liberated and transformed state of being.

Explore the realm within and observe what surfaces for you with this 10-Minute Meditation *Going Deep Within Yourself* by Great Meditation. (*Scan QR code*)

4.28
*Hānameṣāṁ **kleśavaduktaṁ**.*

The removal of these arising **saṁskāras** follows the same process as the **kleśas**.

Patanjali reminds us again and again that our pain and suffering can be removed. How? Through the consistent, persistent practice that is steady and *without* pause.

Through our commitment to our practice, we reach the highest levels of consciousness. *Avidya* ceases and all attachments to worldly experience disappear. The **kleśas** lifted, we hold the keys to freedom of the self from the shackles of pain and suffering.

The practice of yoga is a journey inward—a journey that terminates our suffering by unraveling the knots of physical discomfort, mental anguish, and spiritual discord. In our transformation beyond the eight limbs of yoga, we start to move in rhythm with the ebb and flow of life without becoming consumed by our experience of it. And while the absence of suffering does not mean the absence of challenges, our steady nature enables us to find contentment, even amidst life's trials.

Liberation is not merely a personal triumph. It reflects the shared aspiration of manifesting a world free from the pervasive grip of suffering. Patanjali's vision extends beyond an individual quest for relief; it envisions a collective consciousness marked by compassion, peace, and understanding. Through our individual choices, we have the power to usher in a realm where suffering becomes a distant echo, and humanity exists in harmony as One.

4.29 to 4.32
Dharmamega Samādhi
Cloud of Virtues

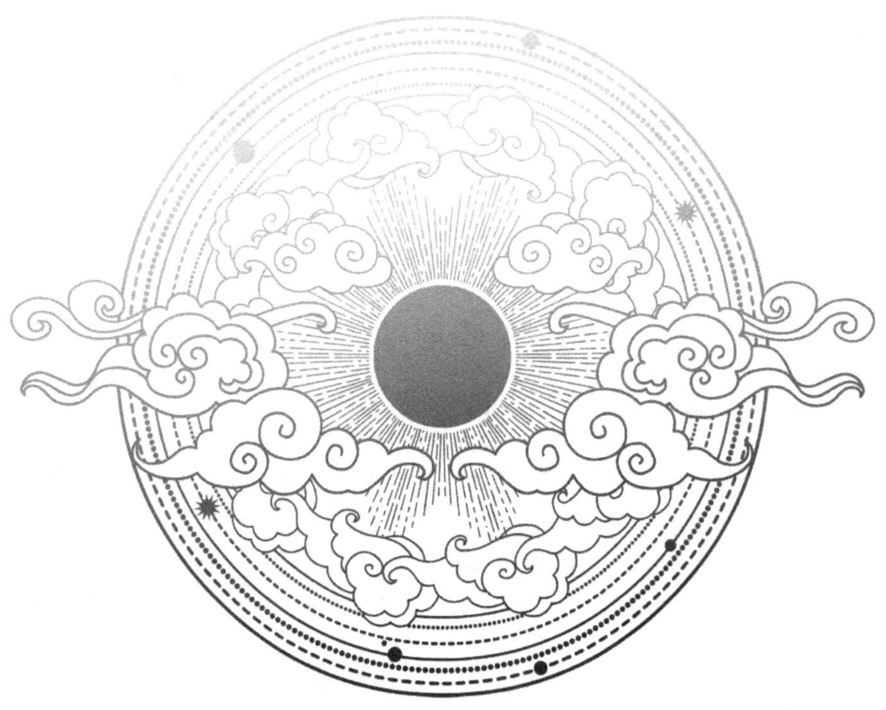

Yoga is the journey of the self, through the self to the Self.
- Bhagavad Gita -

4.29

*Prasaṁkhyāne'pyakusīdasya sarvathā **viveka***
*khyāter**dharmameghḥ samādhiḥ***

No longer interested in the pursuit of even the highest meditation, having reached divine insight **viveka**, arises a state of deep absorption (**samādhi**) known as the 'cloud of virtues' (**dharma-megha**).

After the continuous dedication to *sadhana*, meditation, and the quest for Freedom, the moment arrives when the pursuit of Enlightenment becomes obsolete. Upon releasing all attachments (*vairagya*) to both worldly and spiritual rewards, and understanding the distinction between the Knower (*puruṣa*) and the known (*prakṛti), the yogi crosses* the threshold and transforms into a living, breathing embodiment of Enlightenment itself–**dharmamegha samādhi.**

Just as a cloud pours rain, with *dharmamegha samādhi,* virtues shower upon the yogi from above. With divine awareness and discernment, there is no longer the need for the rewards from the manifest world. The inner world is now the true reward. In every moment, the yogi holds **viveka-jñāna** and with this divine wisdom all ignorance, judgment, bias, jealousy, anger, contempt etc. ceases to exist as do all impurities (**malās**). Unclouded by *kleśas,* the awakened yogi is a living embodiment of *satchitananda*–love, supreme insight, and Bliss.

In the outpouring of virtues, the yogi's *dharma* also becomes clear. The genuine path of the soul is to shine forth love, compassion, and wisdom. Their very presence uplifts and inspires, igniting the spark of divine realization, and serving as a catalyst for the spiritual awakening of others.

Become One with Universal consciousness and join Mooji with *You are Pure Awareness.* (*Scan QR code*)

4.30

*Taṭḥ **kleśa karma** nivṛttiḥ.*

From that (*dharmamegha samādhi*) arises the cessation of suffering (**kleśa**) and the actions that cause suffering (**karma**).

4.31

*Tadā **sarvā**varaṇa**malā**petasya **jñāna**syānantyājjñeyamalpam.*

Then, with the removal of all coverings and impurities (**malās**), the vastness of divine knowledge (**jñāna**) shines forth, leaving only a small portion of the unknown.

After *dharmamegha samādhi* destroys the roots of suffering, the perpetual cycle of *karmic* actions comes to an end. Through this showering of insight, the yogi experiences complete release from the burdens that bind them, and very little is beyond their grasp. Beneath this "cloud of virtues," they have reached the pinnacle of Enlightenment.

The stilled **guṇas** usher in a state of pure *sattvic* awareness. *Sattva*, in its purest form, creates peace in every moment. With every moment alive with clarity, freedom, and supreme wisdom, nothing can shake the yogi. Liberation is now within grasp.

4.32

*Tataḥ kṛtārthānām **pariṇāmakramasamāptirguṇānām**.*

Now, their purpose complete, the transformation of the **guṇas** ceases.

When we rest in our true Nature, the energies of *rajas*, *tamas* and *sattva* are no longer distinct. With the energies lulled, the limitations associated with the **guṇas** are transcended.

To put this simply, all the energies are now in equilibrium, quiet, joyful and balanced. Now actions are driven by a sense of purpose and fulfillment, rather than an insatiable pursuit of desires.

Of course, the forces of energy do not disappear entirely. They continue to spin and move around us, but they no longer entangle us in the web of suffering.

As the dualities of life harmonize, there are no longer extreme shifts between good and bad, high and low, happy and sad. Emotions and experiences find balance. In our profound connection with higher consciousness, instead of feeling separate from the universe, we find Oneness and Divine interconnectedness with all of existence. With the **guṇas** in balance, love stands strong over fear, injustice, hate and discouragement.

In this elevated state of being, the yogi keeps the **guṇas** in abeyance, restraining and using them when necessary. They serve as devoted servants, supporting without imposing, allowing the essence of the Universal Self to shine forth undisturbed.

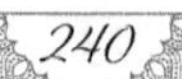

4.33 to 4.34
Kaivalya
Liberation

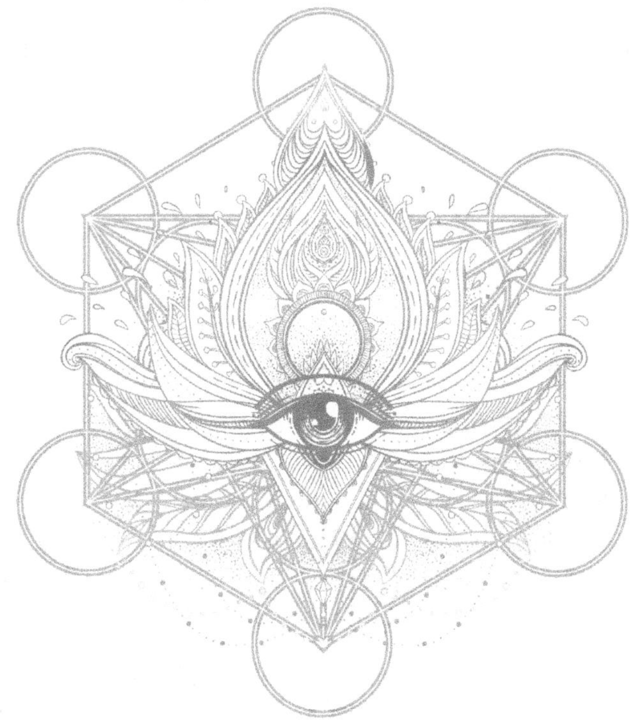

A single drop of the ocean has all the qualities of the ocean.
When a drop meets the ocean, it becomes the ocean.

- Jiddu Krishnamurti -

4.33

*Kṣaṇapratiyogī **pariṇāmā**parāntanirgrāhyaḥ kramaḥ.*

The process of transformation (**pariṇāmā**) is a constant, continuous moment-to-moment flow (**kṣaṇa**); its purpose is impossible to grasp until its end.

As the interplay of the *guṇas* subsides within us, we become more resilient to life's inevitable ups and downs.

Kaivalya brings with it the ability to remain in a state of pure awareness unaffected by the transient fluctuations of our external experiences.

Transcending the fluctuations of these energies, the yogi understands that this "end" of activity of the *guṇas* is really the beginning of Freedom. The yogi, moving effortlessly in a state of pure awareness is freed from the shackles of time and now comprehends that there is *no* beginning and *no* end.

Reaching this culmination, and liberated from the constraints of time, the yogi embraces impermanence and radiates both powerfully and humbily in the essence of divine joy. With this profound realization, the yogi aligns with the perpetual flow of transformation, unfolding their own "best self" in the ever-unfurling tapestry of existence.

4.34

Puruṣārthaśūnyānām guṇānām pratiprasavaḥ kaivalyam
svarūpa pratiṣṭhā vā citiśakter iti

Kaivalya, ultimate liberation, takes place when the forces of nature (**guṇā**s) have served their purpose and revert to their primal state. Freed from the influence of the **guna**s, higher awareness resides in **svarūpa**, one's own essential Nature.

Patanjali has guided us to the pinnacle of our yogic journey—**kaivalya.** He has given us the tools to move from suffering to *sattva* to Freedom. This state of **kaivalya** is beyond thought and word, only to be realized through the complete transformation of consciousness.

In isolation with our *sattvic* spirit, embodying love, divine knowledge and Bliss, we recognize that we are inseparable from the vast ocean of Universal consciousness.

As we conclude this exploration, may you carry the essence of the *Yoga Sūtras* within your heart, embracing the timeless wisdom it holds. May you continue to tread the path to Self-realization, recognizing the eternal *sattva*, the pure Bliss. This Bliss, the *satchitananda*, that is ever present within you is the *same* Bliss that resides within *all* of humanity.

After Thought

The journey of yoga is a process of self-discovery and self-unfoldment. It is a journey of transcending the limitations of the mind and the ego and realizing the infinite potential at the core of our being. When we have reached the end of this journey, when the *puruṣa* within us has reached its purest state, we find that the answers we have been searching for have been within us all along.

As a final note, I encourage you to put down your books and stop searching for answers outside of yourself. Pause and reflect upon the knowledge you have gained and the insights that have unfolded within you. The truth you seek is not in the words of others but within the depths of your own soul. Embrace the silence that envelops you and listen attentively to the voice of your own consciousness. Settle into your own seat and learn from the truth of your being. Here may you find solace, peace, and fulfillment in the light of your own awakened consciousness.

As you step away from these words and immerse yourself in the boundless possibilities of your own existence, may the essence of yoga accompany you, illuminating each step of your path. May you find joy in the discovery of your own truth and embrace the fullness of your being.

I leave you with this beautiful rendition of the following chant sung by the 3Nity Brothers with Gaia Meditation.

Lokah Samastah Sukhino Bhavantu

May all beings be happy and free,
May my dharma, my life's purpose
contribute to that Freedom for all…

(Scan QR code)

Acknowledgments

I extend my gratitude to Rachel Lando, owner of Patient Care Movement for her contributions as the main editor.

Special thanks to Anne Marie Viviene for her poetic final touches with editing. Her expertise and commitment to excellence ensured the manuscript reached its highest potential.

To my book designer and publishing consultant, Katie Mullaly, who was there for me every step of the way. Her unwavering support, professionalism, and dedication were instrumental in bringing this book to fruition. Thank you, Katie!

To Alec Soderberg, for his philosophical guidance, inspirational music, and transcendent voice.

I am also grateful to my friend editors Fatima Doman, Tracey Hausman, Debbi Leuteritz, Nicole Blumin, Shoree Boyd, Margaret Koblasova, Donna Macaleer, and Angela Egner whose feedback and encouragement were instrumental in refining this manuscript. Their insights and perspectives enriched the work immeasurably.

To Alex Jr Paldon owner of AJ Creative Solutions for his exceptional work with the final elements of the book.

I would also like to express my sincere appreciation to those who gave permission to include their videos and meditations. Through this collaboration and weaving together the wisdom and expertise of various contributors, I have been able to bring the ancient teachings of the Yoga Sūtras into practical, everyday use, making this wisdom accessible and applicable to modern life.

And finally to my partner Hanz Johansson, who has supported me through this immense project, every step of the way. His unwavering love kept me believing in myself and this project.

Appendix A

Nine Dṛṣṭi

One
Name: Nāsāgrai Dṛṣṭi
Looking Place: Tip of the nose
Pose Example: Upward Facing Dog (Ūrdhva Mukha Svānāsana)

Two
Name: Bhūmadhyā Dṛṣṭi or Ājñā Dṛṣṭi
Looking Place: Third eye
Pose Examples: Upward Facing Plank (Pūrvottānāsana) and Fish Pose (Matsyāsana)

Three
Name: Nābhi Chakra Dṛṣṭi
Looking Place: Navel
Pose Example: Downward Dog (Adho Mukha Svanāsana)

Four
Name: Hastāgrai Dṛṣṭi
Looking Place: Hand
Pose Example: Triangle Pose (Trikonāsana)

Five
Name: Pādayoragrai Dṛṣṭi
Looking Place: Toes
Pose Examples: Shoulder Stand (Sarvāngāsana) and in most seated forward bending poses

Six

Name: Parśva Dṛṣṭi

Looking Place: Far to the right

Pose Example: Reclining Hand-to Big-Toe Pose (Supta Pādāngusthāsana)

Seven

Name: Parśva Dṛṣṭi

Looking Place: Far to the left

Pose Example: Sage Marichi Pose (Marichyāsana)

Eight

Name: Aṅgustha Madhya Dṛṣṭi

Looking Place: Thumbs

Pose Example: Upward Salute Pose (Ūrdhva Hastāsana)

Nine

Name: Ūrdhva Dṛṣṭi or Antara Dṛṣṭi

Looking Place: Up to the sky

Pose Example: Warrior One (Vīrabhadrāsana I)

Appendix B

Outline of the Stages of Samādhi
(According to Patanjali)*

Samprajñāta Samādhi

Vitarka (Reasoning)
1. Savitarka: Mental functions still occur with concentration on an object.
2. Nirvitarka: Mental alternations cease, revealing subtleties of the object.

Vicāra (Reflection)
3. Savicāra: The mind is submersed in the subtleties of the object.
4. Nirvicāra: Subtle differentiation is relinquished, leading to a sāttvic state.
5. Ānanda (Bliss) Identification with ego stops, bringing rapture and ecstasy.
6. Asmitā (I-Ness) Suppression of Asmitā leads to the perception of a cosmic mind and pure "Is-Ness."

Asamprajñāta Samādhi
7. Dharmamegha Samādhi: This is not necessarily a separate stage and could be considered the equivalent of Asamprajñāta Samādhi. Here the practitioner experiences the "cloud of dharma" or a state of divine knowledge and virtue where all attachments (*vairagya*) to both worldly and spiritual rewards are released.
8. Kaivalya: State of ultimate liberation and union with Universal Consciousness.

*The essence of Samādhi lies in the direct experience of deep meditative absorption, transcending the conceptual framework of stages or categories. Therefore, the number of stages of Samādhi may vary according to different traditions but what remains central is the transformative experience of union with the Divine.

Appendix C

Ananda Ayurveda Health

Learn to live in harmony with your own true nature. Take charge of your health and see your life's fabric differently from the Vedic perspective. If you are interested in a professional Ayurvedic consultation through Ananda Ayurveda LLC scan here:

Constitution Questionnaire

Choose the dominant description of you over the long term when you are healthy and well rested. You may choose more than one answer, if applicable.

SECTION I: Physical Characteristics

1. Physique
   a. I am taller or shorter than average with narrow hips and shoulders.
   b. I am average in height with a moderate build and a tendency toward defined muscles.
   c. I am stocky, broad, with a well-developed physique.

2. Weight
   a. I am thin; my bones (e.g. knuckles) and blood vessels tend to be prominent.
   b. I am of moderate weight. If I gain weight, I can take it off with relative ease.
   c. I am heavy and easily gain weight that only comes off slowly.

3. Hair
   a. My hair is more dry, kinky, brittle, curly, coarse.
   b. My hair is more fine, light color, soft, prone to early graying or balding.
   c. My hair is more thick, oily, wavy, luxurious, coarse, dark color.

4. Skin
   a. My skin is dry, thin and dusty colored.
   b. My skin is oily, moderate thickness, prone to freckles and moles, rosy or ruddy or sallow.
   c. My skin is moist, thick, soft and pale.

5. Eyes
   a. My eyes are small, dry, brown and I tend to blink a lot.
   b. My eyes are sharp, penetrating, deep set, with reddish or yellowish whites.
   c. My eyes are large, attractive, moist, with white whites, brown or deep blue irises.

6. Eyebrows
   a. My brows are narrow with thin hair density, dry, and firm to touch.
   b. My brows are medium.
   c. My brows are thick, bushy, oily, soft.

7. Nose

   a. My nose is small, thin, bumpy, slightly crooked with a thin bridge.
   b. My nose is medium-sized, reddish with large pores.
   c. My nose is large relative to my face, oily, with a wide bridge.

8. Lips

   a. My lips are thin, dry or chapped, narrow and dark.
   b. My lips are medium, soft, pink.
   c. My lips are large, moist, firm and smooth.

9. Teeth

   a. My teeth have at least two of these characteristics: crooked, large or very small, protruding, with large spaces, with receding gums.
   b. My teeth are medium-sized, yellowish.
   c. My teeth are large, straight, and white.

10. Tongue

   a. My tongue is thin with cracks or scallops, dark pink, blue-tinged on undersurface.
   b. My tongue is moderately thick, red-pointed, moist.
   c. My tongue is thick, whitish, lighter pink.

11. Neck

   a. My neck is narrow and long.
   b. My neck is medium.
   c. My neck is thick and strong.

12. Chest
   a. My chest is thin, not muscular; breasts are small (women).
   b. My chest is medium.
   c. My chest is muscular, thick, barrel-shaped, breasts are large (women).

13. Hands
   a. My hands are cold, dry, and well-lined, with veins and knuckles prominent.
   b. My hands are medium, warm, pink, moist, soft.
   c. My hands are large, thick, with smooth knuckles.

14. Calves
   a. My calves are small and firm.
   b. My calves are medium.
   c. My calves are thick and firm.

15. Feet
   a. My feet are small or very large, cold, dry and rough.
   b. My feet are medium-sized, soft, warm, pink.
   c. My feet are large, thick, solid, moist.

16. Hands
   a. My palms are rectangular and I have long narrow fingers.
   b. My palms are square and my finger the same length as my palms.
   c. My palms are square and fleshy and I have short wide fingers.

17. Nails
   a. My nails are dry, small, ridged, crack or chip easily.
   b. My nails are pink, medium thickness and size, soft, oily.
   c. My nails are large, hard, thick.

18. Joints

    a. My joints are thin, prominent, and tend to make cracking sounds.
    b. My joints are medium, soft, loose, and tend to sprain rather than break.
    c. My joints are large, thick and strong.

19. Bones

    a. The relative circumference is small compared to their length.
    b. The relative circumference is medium compared to their length.
    c. The relative circumference is large compared to their length.

20. Face

    a. The shape of my face is long and narrow.
    b. The shape of my face is angular, perhaps with strong jaw and cheekbones.
    c. The shape of my face is round and soft.

21. Facial Energy

    a. My facial energy is subtle and less defined than others.
    b. My facial energy is intense and passionate.
    c. My facial energy is sweet, serene and calm.

22. Pulse

    a. Rapid, thready, thin, undulating.
    b. Bounding, strong, froglike.
    c. Slow, broad, swanlike.

SECTION I TOTAL: a_______   b_______   c_______

SECTION II: Body Functions

23. Appetite
a. Irregular, sometimes I forget to eat, other times I am very hungry between meals.
b. Sharp hunger, dislikes missing meals, can eat large quantities of food.
c. Steady, can miss a meal without discomfort, feels best eating smaller.

24. Digestive Imbalance Tendency
a. I often get gas or bloating after meals.
b. I often get acid or heartburn after meals.
c. I often feel heavy or sleepy after meals.

25. Bowel Movements
a. Hard, dry, dark brown, constipation 1 time/day or less.
b. Loose and soft or diarrhea, abundant, medium brown, regular 2+ times/day.
c. Heavy, slow, thick, regular, pale, large, oily 1 time/day.

26. Urine
a. Frequent small amounts of dark urine.
b. Abundant, deep yellow, clear, occasionally slightly burning.
c. Moderate, concentrated, cloudy.

27. Perspiration
a. Scanty, without strong odor.
b. Profuse, strong odor.
c. Moderate quantity, sweet odor.

28. Physical Activity Pattern
    a. Quick, restless, easily sidetracked.
    b. Focused, intense and efficient, perfectionist dislikes interruptions.
    c. Deliberate calm and steady.

29. Learning Pattern
    a. Quick to learn, quick to forget if not used.
    b. Moderate.
    c. Longer to learn slow to forget.

30. Endurance, Strength, Immunity
    a. Low, tires easily, minor illnesses often.
    b. Moderate, rarely sick, moderate strength.
    c. High, rarely sick, can keep steady on without missing work.

31. Libido
    a. Frequent desire, low stamina.
    b. Moderate desire, passionate.
    c. Cyclical, excellent stamina.

32. Weather Intolerance
    a. Cold temperatures, wind, dryness.
    b. Heat and humidity.
    c. Cold temperatures, dampness.

SECTION II TOTAL: a________   b________   c________

SECTION III: Subtle Body

33. Speech
    a. Talkative, enthusiastic, speaks quickly, can ramble at times, high pitch.
    b. Argumentative, precise, convincing, sharp, direct speech, medium pitch.
    c. Slow, sometimes monotonous, low-pitched, melodious speech.

34. Voice
    a. Low volume, hoarse, vibrato, high pitched.
    b. Sharp, loud, laughing, can project.
    c. Deep, resonant, melodic.

35. Social Temperament
    a. Shy or very outgoing, good storyteller.
    b. Assertive, good leader.
    c. At ease, good listener, companionable.

36. Gait
    a. Quick with short light steps.
    b. Purposeful pace at moderate speed, feet go out in front.
    c. Slow, long strides.

37. Mental Tendencies
    a. Questioning, hypothesizing, can change mind easily, creative, enthusiastic.
    b. Leader, self-motivated, driven. Decides easily but can change with new information.
    c. Stable, logical, slow to make or change decisions.

38. Sleep
    a. Wakes easily, sleeps 5-7 hours per night, tendency toward insomnia, lies awake thinking.
    b. Sound sleeper, 6-8 hours per night. If wakes, gets up and works until sleepy again.
    c. Deep, easy to fall asleep difficult to awaken.

39. Memory
    a. Short, forgets relatively easily.
    b. Average, clear on details.
    c. Long.

40. Emotional State/Tendency when Threatened or Stressed
    a. Unpredictable, fearful, anxious, worried.
    b. Aggressive, irritable, judgmental, uncompromising, suspicious.
    c. Withdraws, ignores, becomes stubborn, may become depressed.

41. Spiritual Life
    a. Irregular.
    b. Disciplined.
    c. Not much interested.

42. Love and Romance
    a. Many romances, falls in and out love easily.
    b. Passionate and intense.
    c. Affectionate, comfortable, likes long term relationships.

43. Dreams
   a. Flying, running, fear, searching, traveling.
   b. Fire, passion, violence, strife, battle.
   c. Romance, water, erotic, emotional.

44. Hygiene
   a. Clean and neat, dislikes disorder.
   b. Functionally clean, according to priorities.
   c. Messy, cluttered at times.

45. Work Habits
   a. Selfless service, often volunteers.
   b. Works intensely toward personal goals.
   c. Procrastinates, but steady when gets going.

46. Leisure
   a. Travel, movies, dancing, parties, socializing.
   b. Sports, reading, projects, hobbies, developing personal talents.
   c. Watching movies, theater, concerts, dining out, television, sleep, sex, food, reading.

47. Financial Behavior
   a. Buys on impulse, dislikes sticking to a budget.
   b. Plans, but enjoys luxuries.
   c. Frugal, but spends money on food and entertainment.

SECTION III TOTAL: a_________   b_________   c_________

GRAND TOTALS ALL SECTIONS

	SECTION I	SECTION II	SECTION III	TOTAL
a				
b				
c				

KEY:
All "A" answers correspond to VATA dosha.
All "B" answers correspond to PITTA dosha.
All "C" answers correspond to KAPHA dosha.

Vata Predominant (mostly "A" answers)

Characteristics: Creative, sensitive, flexible, talkative, enthusiastic, alert, quick moving, social butterfly or very shy, responsible. Can be a strong influencer, dreamer, storyteller.

When out of balance, vata predominant people can be scattered, ungrounded, anxious, constipated, depleted.

Vata dosha is aggravated by winds and drafts, excessive movement and travel, excessive chaos, noise, intense feelings/sensations, cold dry weather, overwork, mental strain, irregular schedules, especially irregular mealtimes and sleep times.

Vata predominant people do best with regular mealtimes and sleep routines. Their food is best warm, moist and heavy. They may enjoy heavy soft blankets on their beds at night. Moisture and oiling the skin calms the nervous system as well as counteracting dryness. Taking time to rest and relax is essential.

Vata predominant people thrive with the development of faith and self-confidence.

Pitta Predominant (mostly "B" answers)

Characteristics: Pitta predominant people are visionary, intelligent, articulate and focused. Their courage and practical, goal-oriented outlook makes them exceptional leaders. They enjoy competition, even with themselves. They are warm and compassionate when in balance.

When their pitta nature is out of balance, they become hot and intense. This includes becoming physically hot, experiencing hot emotions such as frustration, impatience, irritation and anger. Their intensity may carry a sharp quality. They can become judgmental rather than compassionate.

Pitta dosha is aggravated by all things that increase heat: pressure, excessive sun, excessively spicy/pungent/salty foods, alcohol, smoking, friction.

Pitta predominant people do best with cool weather and cool water. Moonlight, softness, humor and acceptance are all good remedies for excessive pitta dosha.

Pitta predominant people thrive with the development of self-acceptance and compassion.

Kapha Predominant (mostly "C" answers)

Characteristics: Stable, sturdy, methodical, slow, enduring, strong, loyal, affectionate, companionable, slow to react.

When their kapha nature is out of balance, kapha dominant people can become stubborn, dull, possessive, stuck and/or indulgent. They may oversleep, overeat, or avoid stimulation with excessive routine.

Kapha dosha is aggravated by damp and cold, too little variety and stimulation, a sedentary lifestyle, heavy cold or fatty foods and overindulgence in eating and/or sleeping.

Kapha predominant people do best with variety that is introduced slowly, easing around their resistance. All activity eases excess kapha. Spicy food, spontaneity, giving things away are all remedies for excessive kapha. Kapha predominant people thrive when performing selfless service.

Dual Doshas:

Often two of the doshas are close to equally presenting in a constitution. Simply blend the characteristics listed accordingly to describe vata-pitta, vata-kapha, pitta-kapha predominant people.

Appendix D

Sutras by Subject - English

Sutras by Subject - Sanskrit

Mantras, Chants, Hindu Gods

Chakra Bija Mantras 3.39

Chakra Mantras 3.30

Chandra (moon) Mantra 4.22 (Om Shram Shreem Shroum Sah Chandramasé Namah)

Ganesh 3.25 (Om Gam Ganapataye Namaha)

Gayatri Mantra 3.29 (Oṃ bhūḥ bhuvaḥ svaḥ tat savitur vareṇyaṃ bhargo devasya dhīmahi dhiyo yo naḥ pracodayāt)

Hanuman 3.24 (Om Ham Hanumate Namah)

Indra 3.47

Karuna Mantra - After Thought (Lokah Samastah Sukhino Bhavantu)

Lakshmi 3.41 (Om Shreem Maha Lakshmi Namaha)

Saraswati 3.55 (Om Shreem Hreem Saraswatyai Namaha)

Shiva 1.29, 2.44 (Om Namah Shivaya)

Appendix E

Chakra Outline

FIRST CHAKRA – Mūlādhāra (Root Chakra)

Mantra: *I am always safe, rooted and grounded from the center of my being*
Location: Pelvic floor, perineum
Element: Earth
Color: Red
Seed mantra: LAM
Frequency: 396 HZ
When balanced: Groundedness and feelings of safety and security
Out of Balance: Fearfulness, may eat too much or too little
Yoga postures: Any pose that feels a connection to the earth, hip openers
Gemstone: Ruby
Yantra: Circle with four petals with a downward-pointing triangle
Sense: Smell

SECOND CHAKRA – Svādhiṣṭhāna (Sacral Chakra)

Mantra: *I flow with the rhythms of life*
Location: Below the navel
Element: Water
Color: Orange
Bija (Seed) mantra: VAM
Frequency: 417 HZ
When balanced: Emotional and sexual well-being
Out of balance: Trouble with intimacy and emotions
Yoga postures: Hips, vinyasa flow
Gemstone: Coral, Amber
Yantra: White/silver crescent moon with four petals
Sense: Taste

THIRD CHAKRA – Maṇipūra (Solar Plexus)

Mantra: *I stand in my personal power*
Location: Solar plexus
Element: Fire
Color: Yellow
Bija (Seed) sound: RAM
Frequency: 528 HZ
When balanced: Healthy self-esteem
Out of balance: Social issues, digestion problems
Yoga postures: Twists, standing postures, core
Gemstone: Amber, gold
Yantra: Inverted triangle with a T-shape on its three sides, ten petals
Sense: Sight

FOURTH CHAKRA – Anāhata (Heart Chakra)

Mantra: *I open my heart fully to all with unconditional love*
Location: Heart
Element: Air
Color: Green
Seed mantra: YAM
Frequency: 639 HZ
When balanced: Unconditional love
Out of balance: Depression, pessimism, respiratory problems
Yoga postures: Backbends, lateral bends
Gemstone: Emerald
Yantra: Hexagram with two interlaced triangles, twelve petals
Sense: Touch

FIFTH CHAKRA – Viśuddha (Throat Chakra)

Mantra: *I follow and speak my truth*
Location: Throat
Element: Space, ether
Color: Blue
Seed mantra: HAM
Frequency: 741 HZ
When balanced: Easy, clear communication
Out of balance: Speech/thyroid issues
Yoga postures: Using voice, throat openers
Gemstone: Turquoise, topaz
Yantra: Circle with a full white moon, sixteen petals
Sense: Auditory

SIXTH CHAKRA – Ājñā (The Master Chakra)

Mantra: *I follow my intuition, the path of Truth*
Location: Third-eye center
Element: Includes all elements
Color: Violet
Seed sound: OM
Frequency: 852 HZ
When balanced: Calm and focused
Out of balance: Confusion about one's spiritual path, problems with senses
Yoga Postures: Balance postures with drishti
Gemstone: Sapphire
Yantra: A circle with an inverted triangle and above the triangle a shiva lingam or astral body, two petals
Sense: 6th sense

SEVENTH CHAKRA – Sahasrāra (Thousand Petal Lotus)

Mantra: *A greater spirit connects me to all that I do*
Location: The crown of the head and beyond
Element: Beyond the elements
Color: Violet and crystalline light
Bija Seed sound: AH
Frequency: 963 HZ
When balanced: Unity Consciousness
Out of balanced: Spiritual separation
Yoga postures: Wheel pose, savasana, inversions such as headstand
Gemstone: Amethyst, diamond
Yantra: Beyond with a thousand petals
Sense: Universal Consciousness

Appendix F

Catalogue of Practices

Pada 1

1.3   *I Am That*, Nisargadatta Maharaj

1.4   *Smile Guided Meditation*, Tara Brach (10:00)

1.5   *Lake Meditation*, Jon Kabat-Zinn (MBSR) (13:00)

1.6   *Clear Your Mind from Overthinking*, Great Meditation (8:00)

1.7   *Power to Discern*, Inner Space Meditation (3.31)

1.8   *Guided Meditation: Transforming Fear*, Tara Brach (12:00)

1.9   *Guided Body Awareness Meditation*, Dr. Arielle Schwartz (9:42)

1.10 *Bone Deep Sleep*, Jennifer Piercy, Insight Timer (15:00)

1.11 *Healing Past Trauma*, davidji (15:40)

1.12 *Prana Vinyasa*, Shiva Rea (1:00.00)

1.13 *Ashtanga Yoga Primary Series*, Pattabhi Jois (1:18:07)

1.14 *Sankalpa Guided Meditation*, Shilpa Lewis, Omni Mindfulness (14:56)

      Spark Your Sankalpa guided suggestions, Shilpa Lewis

      By utilizing Shilpa's guided meditation and accompanying informational graphic as a reference for the representation of sūtras, Susan of Yoga Awakening acknowledges and agrees to attribute credit to Shilpa as the author of the guided meditation and graphic. This ac-

knowledgement must include a reference to Shilpa's website and her name. Any use of the guided meditation or graphic without proper attribution is strictly prohibited.

1.15 *Detachment (Vairāgya),* Max Baker Yoga (8:00)

1.16 *Explore the Gunas Meditation,* Susan Fendler

Exploring the Gunas Yoga Practice, Shiloh

1.18 *She Let Go,* by Safire Rose, read by John Siddique, (2.39)

1.19 *The Art of Happiness,* Dalai Lama

1.20 *Most Powerful Meditation on Faith,* Positive Magazine (10:00)

1.22 *Morning Routine REVEALED For Success!* (4:08)
DE Stress with Mindful Meditation, Jay Shetty (10:08)

1.23 Bhakti Fest Song and Dance, Rishikesh, India by Mooji Music (1:43:14)

1.27 *Ohm* Spotify playlist, Yoga Awakening

1.29 *Daily Japa Meditation,* Braydon Mackenzie, Insight Timer (17:00)

1.32 8-Week Free Mindfulness Based Meditation Stress Reduction Program (MBSR)

1.33 *5-Minute Loving Kindness Meditation, Unearth Compassion* (5:00)

1.34 *Square (box) Breathing,* UAB Student Affairs (3:18)

1.35 *Sensory Awareness Meditation,* Meditations and Soundscapes (12:58)

1.36 *Jyothi (light) Meditation,* Adeline108 (10:23)
Light House, Spotify, MC Yogi
Light of Your Grace, Mooji Baba

1.37   *Peace is Every Step* by Thich Nhat Hanh

1.38   *Calming Yoga Nidra*, Tamara Skyhawk (Verma) (14:42)

1.39   *Flower – Fresh*, Thich Nhat Hanh (11:04)

1.40   *I Am the Universe*, davidji (15:00)

1.41   *Illusion Itself is Illusory*, Samaneri Jayasāra (20:00) The link to the reading has been given with the uploader's permission and that Samaneri Jayasara (as a Buddhist nun) does not profit from nor commercialize her work.

1.42   *Meditation: Candle Gazing*, Susi Amendola, Insight Timer (7:31)

1.43   *Anahata Dharana Meditation*, Yog se Yogyata (15:00)

1.44   *Binaural Beats Theta Waves Meditation*, Great Meditation (11:02)

1.45   *Boundless Ocean*, from the Ashtavakra Gita, The I AM Project (11:42)

1.49   *The Immensity of Being*, Mooji (4.53)

Pada 2

2.2   *Paramnansa Yogananda's Energization Exercises*, Ananda Sangha Mumbai (16:34)

2.3   *The 5 Kleshas (Poisons)*, Yoga Philosophy Explained, Shivatman Yoga (8:41)

2.6   *Do We Need an Ego?* Lecture by Anand Ji, Sattva Connect (7-day free trial) (25:16)
How to Tell When Ego Is Running Your Life (and What to Do Instead), Alignment with Veronica (19:25

2.7 *Let Go and Let Love*, Integrative Practice, Anand Ji (7-day free trial) (1:17:47)
Yoga Flow To Release Everything, Empty Your Mind... Be Water, My Friend, Boho Beautiful (26:18)

2.8 *Dealing with Avoidance*, Marcus L. Petersen, in collaboration with Brian from Metaverse (22:36)

2.9 *Guided Death Meditation to Live More* (Maranasati), The Downward Doug (21:19)

2.11 *5 Minute Mindfulness Meditation*, Sherri Lukac, Red House Wellness. (5:00)

2.12 *Egoic Mantra, Daniel Roquéo,* Insight Timer (11:00)

2.13 *Permission to Let Go,* Mindful Movement (23:00)

2.14 *Remember to Choose Love!* Great Meditation (10:40)

2.15 *Release Negative Energy and End Suffering* (Buddhism) by davidji (22:30)

2.17 *Rewrite the Past*, Sattva Connect (7-day free trial) (1:06:55)

2.19 *Cellular Breathing in the Bones*, Mark Taylor, Insight Timer (21:21)

2.20 *Awareness*, Ram Das, Spotify (17:00)

2.21 *The Lotus Flower Meditation*, Braydon Mackenzie (20:00)

2.22 *Wisdom Mantra – Om Mani Padme Hum, Ekhartyoga (12:56)*
Om Mani Padme Hum by Shankara – Yoga Vidya Ashram Bad Meinberg (8.28)

2.26 *Silent Yin Yoga For Deep Somatic Release To Soften Into The Heart*, The Bare Female (44:00)

Intermediate *for Shoulders and Upper back*, Yoga Awakening, (40:00)
Advanced / Intermediate Yoga Flow, Boho Beautiful (22.20)

2.28 *Hatha Yoga: Surya Namaskar -Sun Salutation*, Shiva Das (10:44)

2.33 *5 Minute Guided Meditation for Gratitude*, Mindful Movement (5:00)

2.34 *Ahimsa Meditation*, 365 Days of Meditation (9:36)

2.35 *Buddhist Loving Kindness Meditation*, Yoga Awakening with Sue (3:00)

2.37 *Prāṇāyāma & Meditation with Sound Vibrations For Asteya*, Sarah Margaret, Insight Timer (50:00)

2.38 *Nadi Shodhana Prāṇāyāma*, Yoga with Adriene (11:15)

2.39 *Practice Extended Exhale*, Head Space (2.55)

2.40 TrigunaYoga.net

2.41 *How to Detoxify with Kapalabhati*, Akhandā Yoga Institute (6:40)

2.42 *The Divine Romance*, Paramahansa Yogananda

2.43 *Creating Peace from the Inside Out*, 21-Day Meditation, Oprah and Deepak

2.44 *Hare Om Shivaya*, Michael Cohen (8:40)
Om Namah Shivaya, Krishna Das (15.31)

2.46 *Restorative Yoga*, Boho Beautiful (19:53)
Total Body Yoga, Deep Stretch, Yoga With Adriene (45:13)
Energetic Flow, Dice lida-Klein, Glo.com (7-day free trial)

2.47 *Tai Chi Yoga*, SRMD Yoga (45:00)

2.48 *Nondual Guided Meditation*, Shamash (20:00)

2.49   Mindful Breathing to Reconnect with Your Authentic Strengths, Fatima Doman (3:00)

2.50   *Breath* by James Nestor
The Science of Breath by Swami Rama
The Yoga of Breath by Richard Rosen
The Breathing Book by Donna Farhi
Body by Breath by Jill Miller

2.51   *Awakening Cosmic Consciousness*, Anand Ji, SattvaConnect.com (40:38)

2.52   *10 Minute Morning Breathwork Routine, The Key To Happiness*, Breath with Sandy (10:00)

2.53   *15 Minutes Prāṇāyāma*, SRMD (15:45)

2.55   *Humming Bee Breath, Technique-Bhramari Prāṇāyāma*, Sikana English (2:08)

Pada 3

3.2   *I Love You Positive Affirmation Repeated*, Ash Hamilton

3.3   OM playlist, Yoga Awakening, Spotify

3.4   *Yin Yoga To Go Inward & Retreat | Healing Frequency in 432 Hz*, The Bare Female (27:54)
Yoga for Deep Focus, Patrick Beach (24:25)

3.5   *Inner Light Breathing- Meditation*, Cory Cochiolo, Insight Timer (15:57)

3.6   *You are Silence Itself*, Mooji (16:22)

3.8   *Pure Awareness I Am*, Mooji (10:34)

3.11 *Caterpillar to Butterfly Meditation*, Planet Meditation (10:23)

3.12 *Explore Shiva dancing in the Cosmos with The Gods of Yoga - Full Yoga Class Inspired by Lord Shiva - Warrior Flow*, Megan at Yogatrotter, (32:36)

3.15 *I Did Yoga Every Day for Three Years, This is What Happened*, Caro Arevalo (6:53)

3.23 *Chakra Balansing Meditation and Music*, High Vibe Meditation (17:16)
       Awaken the Chakras, Yoga Awakening with Sue (40:00)

3.24 *Hanuman Bolo*, Janin Devi and Andre Maris (duet)
       Hanuman Bolo Dj Drez and Janet Stone

3.25 *Om Gam Ganapataye Namaha*, Gaia Meditation (8:00)
       Power Yoga, Strong Core, by Dig Yoga (16.40)

3.26 *You Are the Cosmos*, Great Meditation (10:06)

3.29 *Light of your Grace* (Gayatri Mantra), Sam Garrett and Mollie Mendoza

3.30 *Awaken the Chakras*, Yoga Awakening with Sue, (42:21)

3.30 *Solar Plexus Chakra Meditation*, Jessica Heslop (10:00)

3.32 *Kurma Nadi: The Tortoise Meditation*, Tony Murdock (9:47)

3.33 *Third Eye & Crown Chakra Activation*, Manifesto Meditations (22:10)
3.35 *Heart Chakra Healing*, Lotus Creek (15:00)

3.37 *5 Senses Guided Imagery*, Dr. Jennifer Andrews (8:55)

3.39 *Chakra Seed Mantra Meditation*, 3Nity Brothers, Gaia Meditation (21:00)
       "Astronomy in India: A Historical Perspective" by B. V. Subbarayappa

3.41 *The Five Vayus,* Movement Meditation (9:00)
Lakshmi (I Choose to Live in Love) – Live in Zürich 2023, Sam Garrett
(9:00)

3.47 *Tibetan Thunderbolt (Dorje) Indestructible Diamond* (19:21)
Sunreed Instruments, Sunreed.com

3.49 *Seeing Without Eyes, Knowing Without Mind,* Mooji (10:47)

3.53 *Leaves on a Stream,* Not Another Meditation (5:07)

3.55 *The Seed Activation,* Niccolò Angeli, Kyrian (37:50)
Saraswati Mahalo, Daphne Tse

Pada 4

4.1 *Ram Das, Going Home,* Netflix

4.3 *50 Minute Yoga Class - Lotus Flow,* Floating Yoga School, (50:00)

4.4 *Effortless Presence,* Anand Ji, SattvaConnect.com (7-day free trial)
(1:14:00)

4.5 *The Power of Now,* Eckhart Tolle
Mindfulness in Plain English, Bhante Gunaratana

4.6 *Be the Witness,* The Mindful Movement (24:24)

4.10 *Discovering Freedom,* Mooji (35:11)

4.11 *Rise of the Phoenix,* Dakota Earth Cloud Walker, Insight Timer (29:37)

4.14 *Earthly Diversity,* Megan Shirey, Insight Timer (10:58)

4.16 *Taking a Shamanic Journey,* Brian Scott (41:12)

Glossary of Sanskrit Words

Abhiniveśa: Clinging to life or fear of death.

Abhyāsa: Practice, specifically referring to the effort to remain absorbed in concentration.

Agamah: Refers to verbal testimony or scriptural authority.

Ahamkara: Ego or the individual sense of self, separate from the true Self.

Ahaṅkāra: Ego or the sense of "I-ness."

Ahimsa: Non-violence, avoidance of harm to all living beings.

Ājñā: The third eye chakra, located in the forehead between the eyebrows, associated with intuition, insight, and inner wisdom.

Ākāśa: Space or the sky.

Akliṣṭa: Sanskrit for "not painful" or "unafflicted." Refers to mental fluctuations (vṛittis) devoid of suffering.

Ākṛṣṇa: Impure or dark, contrasting with purity.

Alinga: That which is unmanifested, potential Prakṛti

Ālokḥ: Light or illumination, often used metaphorically to represent spiritual enlightenment or insight.

Anahata: The heart chakra, situated in the chest area, associated with the element air and related to love, compassion, and emotional balance.

Ananda: Absorption in bliss.

Anastam: Not lost or preserved, the opposite of "nastam."

Āṅgā: Limbs or components, often referring to various aspects or stages.

Antarāyā: Obstacles or disturbances.

Anumāna: A source of valid knowledge, where conclusions are drawn based on reasoning and evidence.

Apana: One of the five vital airs or winds, responsible for downward and eliminative functions.

Aparigraha: Non-possessiveness or non-greed, avoiding the accumulation of unnecessary material possessions.

Āpuṇya: Painful or non-virtuous actions and their results.

Artha: Meaning or significance, often associated with the understanding of an object or word.

Āsana: Physical practice or posture in yoga.

Asmitā: Egoism or the identification with the self.

Asteya: Non-stealing or refraining from theft.

Atman: the eternal, unchanging, and divine essence of an individual.

Aushadhi: Herbs or medicinal plants, often used in traditional medicine systems.

Avasthā: State or condition.

Avidyā: Unawareness or ignorance, often seen as the root of suffering.

Aviśeṣa: The unparticularized; that which forms the subtle qualities of Prakṛti that stem from the self (Ahaṁkāra), including elements such as sound, touch, sight, taste, or smell.

Bandha: A lock or specific muscular engagement used in yoga to direct the flow of energy and enhance physical and energetic alignment.

Bhakti Yoga: A path of yoga focused on devotion to the divine.

Bhava: Refers to the essence of being, inner experiences, or emotional disposition in yoga and spiritual contexts.

Bhāvanātaḥ: Through meditation or contemplation.

Bhoga: Enjoyment or the experience of pleasure, often referring to sensory or material pleasures.

Buddhi: The faculty of intellect, understanding, or discernment.

Bhūmi: Stage or level, often used to describe the various stages or levels of progress in a practice or discipline.

Bhūta: Element or constituent.

Bīja: Seed or source.

Brahmacharya: Celibacy, self-restraint, or moderation.

Buddhi: Intellect or the faculty of understanding.

Candre: Moon or lunar, related to the moon.

Citta: Mind or consciousness.

cittavṛtti: Mental modifications or thought waves.

Darśana: Insight or deep understanding leading towards Self-realization.

Deśa: Place or location.

Deśa-Bandha: The binding or fixing of one's attention to a specific place or point.

Deśair: Place or location.

Dhāraṇā: Concentration, the practice of focusing the mind on a single point or object.

Dharma: Righteousness, duty, or moral and ethical principles.

Dharma-megha: Cloud of virtue or righteousness, symbolizing spiritual transformation.

Dharmin: One who possesses qualities or attributes.

Dhyāna: Meditation, a state of focused awareness and mental absorption.

Dhyānajam: Born of meditation or contemplation.

Dirgha: Prolonged or extended.

Draṣṭṛ: The Seer, often referring to the pure, witnessing consciousness.

Dṛṣṭi: Gaze or focused gaze, used in yoga asanas to enhance concentration and alignment.

Dṛśyam: That which is seen or perceived, often referring to objects of perception.

Dṛśyayoḥ: Of the material world or the objects of perception.

Duḥkhā: Suffering or pain.

Dvandvā: Pairs of opposites or dualities, often referring to contrasting experiences or conditions in life, such as pleasure and pain, gain and loss, or success and failure.

Eka: One or single.

Ekāgratā: One-pointedness or concentration.

Ekāgrya: One-pointedness or the state of focused concentration.

Grahaṇa: The act of meditation.

Grahītṛ: The perceiver or meditator, the one who grasps or apprehends.

Grāhyeṣu:: The object of perception or meditation.

Guna: Three fundamental qualities or energies that exist in everything in the universe.

Guru: A spiritual teacher or guide.

Hasti: Elephant.

Hetu: Cause or reason, often used in philosophical contexts.

Himsa: Violence or harm.

Indriyas: The senses or sensory organs, through which perception and interaction with the external world occur.

Īśvara: The Supreme Being or Universal Consciousness.

Īśvara-praṇidhānā: Surrender to or devotion to Īśvara.

Janma: Previous births or incarnations, referring to past lives.

Jāti: Birth or caste, referring to social or biological categorization.

Jātya: By birth or by caste.

Jñāna: Knowledge or wisdom, often of a spiritual nature.

Jyotiṣmatī: Brilliant luminosity.

Kaivalya: The ultimate state of liberation and aloneness where the individual soul (Atman) realizes its complete independence and unity with the universal consciousness, transcending all limitations and dualities.

Kāla: Time or duration.

Kaṇṭha: Throat or neck.

Karma: Action or deed, associated with the law of cause and effect.

Karmasayo: The repository of past actions and their impressions in the mind.

Karmendriyas: The organs of action including hands, feet, speech, excretion, and reproduction.

karuna: Compassion and empathy toward the suffering of others

Kleśa: Afflictions or sources of suffering referred to as the five kleśas in yoga.

Kliṣṭa: Painful or afflicted.

Kramā: Sequence or order.

Kriyā: Action or activity.

Kriyā Yoga: The path of action to enlightenment, which includes intense practice (tapas), self-study (svādhyāya), along with the study of yogic texts, and surrender to a higher power (iśvara-praṇidhānā).

Kṣaṇa: A moment or an extremely short duration of time.

Kumbhaka: Breath retention or the pause between inhalation and exhalation in prāṇāyāma practice.

Kūrma: Tortoise.

Lakṣaṇa: Characteristics or attributes, often used in the context of identifying qualities.

Lakṣaṇā: Sign or characteristic.

Liṅga: Manas; That which manifests directly from buddhi such as the intellect and logic.

Mahābhūtas: The five great elements representing the fundamental building blocks of the material world. They are Earth (Prithvi), Water (Jala), Fire (Agni), Air (Vayu), and Space (Akasha).

Mahat: Cosmic intelligence, representing the highest level of consciousness.

Mahā-videhā: An advanced state of consciousness where the physical body is no longer a limitation.

Maitrī: Loving-kindness or friendliness.

Malas: Impurities or stains, often referred to in the context of purifying the mind.

Mana: Mind or the thinking faculty.

Maṇipūra: The solar plexus chakra, located in the upper abdomen, associated with the element fire and related to personal power and self-esteem.

Mano: Mind or mental.

Mantra: A word, phrase, or sound that is repeated as a form of meditation, prayer, or spiritual practice.

Maya: Illusion or deceptive power that veils the true nature of reality.

Moksha: Liberation or ultimate spiritual freedom.

Mudita: Joy and happiness experienced in response to the well-being and success of others.

Mūlādhāra: The root chakra, located at the base of the spine, associated with the element earth and related to basic survival instincts.

Nābhi: Navel or abdomen.

Nastam: Lost or destroyed.

Nidra: Sleep.

Nirbīja: Without seed or object, often used to describe a state of meditation where the mind is free from all thoughts and impressions.

Nirvicāra: A stage of meditation without reflection, where the mind is free from mental constructs or thoughts.

Niyama: Observances or ethical principles in yoga philosophy.

OM or Praṇavaḥ: A sacred sound symbolizing the divine vibration that pervades all of creation.

Pada: A chapter or section of a text.

Pañcha: Five.

Pariṇāma: Transformation or change.

Phalā: Fruit or result, referring to the consequences of actions.

Prachchhardnana: Controlled exhalation, a technique in yoga involving regulated breath release.

Prajñā: Wisdom or deep insight, associated with profound spiritual understanding.

Prakāśa: Light or illumination.

Prakṛti: Nature or the material world.

Pramāṇa: Right knowledge or valid means of knowledge through sense perception, logic, and verbal testimony.

Prāṇa: Vital life force or energy, often associated with the breath and the flow of energy within the body.

Prāṇāyāma: Control of breathing techniques in yoga.

Prarabdha: The Sanskrit term for "ripe" or "fructifying." It refers to the portion of one's past karma that has started to bear fruit and is being experienced in the present life. It represents the destiny or life situations one is currently undergoing due to past actions.

Prasāda: Clarity, purity, or a state of grace and tranquility.

Pratipakṣa Bhāvanam: Cultivating opposite or counteractive thoughts or attitudes to overcome negative mental patterns or emotions.

Pratyāhāra: Letting go of sensory distractions or sensory withdrawal, withdrawing the senses from external stimuli.

Pratyakṣa: Sanskrit for "sense perception." It is one of the three sources of valid knowledge in Indian philosophy, involving direct sensory perception of the external world.

Pratyaya: Mental modification, thought, or cognition, often used to describe the content or fluctuations of the mind.

Puṇyā: Pleasurable or virtuous actions and their results.

Pūraka: Inhalation or the act of taking a breath in.

Puruṣa: The pure, unchanging eternal essence of the Self.

Puruṣayor: Of the individual souls or beings.

Rāga: Attachment or desire for pleasurable experiences.

Rechaka: Exhalation or the act of expelling breath.

Śabda: Sound or word, a source of knowledge through verbal testimony.

Sabhīja: With seed or object.

Sahasrāra: The crown chakra, positioned at the top of the head, associated with spiritual connection, enlightenment, and consciousness.

Samādhi: Enlightenment or meditative absorption, the state of profound spiritual realization and oneness with the universe.

Samana: One of the five vital airs, responsible for assimilation and balance.

Samāpata: Complete meditation, absorption.

Saṁskārās: Mental impressions or imprints left in the mind from past experiences or actions.

Saṁtoṣā: Contentment, being satisfied with what one has.

Saṁyama: A combined practice of concentration (Dhāraṇā), meditation (Dhyāna), and absorption (Samādhi) used to gain deep insights, control over mind and body, and develop various powers or abilities.

Saṁyogaḥ: Union or conjunction, often used to describe the coming together or association of two or more things or entities.

Sankalpa: An intention, resolution, or heartfelt commitment made during meditation or yoga practice, aligning one's thoughts and actions with a specific purpose or goal.

Saṅkhyā: Count or number.

Sarva: All or everything.

Sārva-bhaumā: All-pervading or omnipresent.

Sarva-jñātṛtvam: Omniscience or the state of being all-knowing.

Sattva: A state of purity, balance, and harmony in the mind, associated with qualities such as peace, joy, and clarity.

Satya: Truthfulness, honesty, and integrity.

Saucha: Purity or cleanliness, both external and internal.

Savicāra: A stage of meditation with reflection or mental analysis.

Siddha: Accomplished or perfected being.

Siddhis: Accomplishments or supernatural abilities that are attained through the practice of yoga and meditation.

Smayā: Smile or laughter.

Smṛti: Memory.

Śraddhā: Deep faith and trust in spiritual or religious practices.

Sthira: Steadiness or stability, referring to mental and emotional composure and unwavering focus.

Sthūla: Physical or gross. The coarse or tangible aspect of reality, often used to describe the physical body or material existence.

Sukhā: Pleasurable or joyful.

Sūkṣma: Subtle or subtlest, referring to the subtle aspects of existence.

Śūnya: Empty or void, often used in the context of meditation and spiritual philosophy to refer to a state of emptiness or nothingness.

Sūrye: Sun or solar, related to the sun.

Sūtra: A concise and aphoristic statement or verse, often found in ancient Indian texts, typically short and presented in a thread-like fashion.

Svādhiṣṭhāna: The sacral chakra, situated in the lower abdomen, associated with the element water and related to emotions, creativity, and sexuality.

Svādhyāya: Self-study, often involving the study of yogic texts for self-improvement and self-realization.

Svarūpa: One's true or inherent nature.

Svitarkā: With reflection.

Tanmātras: The subtle essence of perception associated with each of the five Mahābhūtas (great elements). They are sound (śabda), touch (sparśa), form or shape (rūpa), taste (rasa), and smell (gandha). Tanmātras represent the subtle aspects of the material world that the senses perceive.

Tapas: Intense practice or discipline, often involving physical, mental, or spiritual austerity.

Tattvas: The fundamental principles or categories that make up the universe. These principles encompass aspects of reality, existence, and consciousness.

Udana: One of the five vital airs, responsible for upward movements and speech.

Upeksa: Equanimity and impartiality, often associated with maintaining emotional balance in the face of life's ups and downs.

Vairāgya: Detachment or dispassion.

Vajra: Thunderbolt or diamond.

Vāsanā: Impressions or latent tendencies in the mind (personality traits).

Vibhuti: Extraordinary or supernatural powers and manifestations attained through advanced spiritual practices.

Vicāra: Concentration on a subtle object.

Vidhāraṇa-ābhyāṁ: Retaining the breath, a breath control technique in yoga.

Vikalpa: Conception or mental construction, a state of imagination in the mind.

Vikṣepa: Distractions or wandering thoughts of the mind.

Viniyogh: Application or practical use, often used in the context of applying knowledge or techniques in a specific way.

Viparyaya: False knowledge or incorrect understanding.

Vīrya: Vigor, mental and physical strength, or effort.

Viṣaya: Qualities of an object or senses.

Viśeṣā: The particularized; that (Tattvas) which serves as the foundation of our perceived world. This includes gross elements of Prakṛti such as earth, water, fire, or air.

Vitarka: Focus on a physical object, or initial thought or analysis.

Viveka: Discrimination or discernment, often referring to the ability to distinguish between the real and the unreal.

Vṛittis: The fluctuations or activities of the mind, including thoughts, emotions, and mental patterns.

Vyana: One of the five vital airs, responsible for circulation and distribution.

Yama: Moral and ethical principles in yoga philosophy.

Yantra: Geometric or symbolic diagrams used in meditation and spiritual practices to focus the mind and represent aspects of the divine.

Yoga: The union of mind, body, and spirit for mental and physical well-being.

Simple Guide to Sanskrit Pronunciation

16 Vowels:

(3 are rare and not included here)

a p*u*p	**ā** f*a*ther
i m*i*t	**ī** m*ee*t
u p*u*t	**ū** f*oo*d
ṛ /ri r*i*d	
e h*ey*	**ai** h*igh*
o h*oe*	**au** h*ow*
aṁ s*um*	**aḥ** echo of the preceding vowel

Consonants:

Gutteral: **k** *k*id   **kh** wor*kh*orse   **g** *go*   **gh** do*gh*ouse   **ṅ** si*ng*

Palatal: **c** /ch *ch*urch   **ch**/chh chur*ch*hill   **j** *j*ump   **jh** lo*dgeh*ouse   **ñ** pi*n*ata

Cerebral: **ṭ** *t*omato   **ṭh** an*th*ill   **ḍ** *d*art   **ḍh** har*dh*eaded   **ṇ** u*n*der

Dental: **t** *w*ater   **th** *Th*ailand   **d** *d*ough   **dh** a*dh*ere   **n** *n*o

Labial: **p** *p*in   **ph** u*ph*ill   **b** *b*ut   **bh** a*bh*or   **m** *m*other

Consonants Simplified:

1. An "h" following a consonant indicates aspiration of the consonant.
2. "**c**" is pronounced "ch" as in "church" (eg, citta - chitta)
3. Nasal sounds are shaped by the following consonants, and thus the pronunciation usually not a problem.
4. "**v**" can sound like *v* or *w* (vayu or swami)
5. "**jn**" sounds like *gya*

Semi Vowels:

y yes   **r** *run*   **l** *lug*   **v** *vodka*

Sibilants:

ś /sh *shawl*   **ṣ**/sh *shine*   **s** *sun*   **h** *hot*

Compound Consonants:

kṣ/ksh *actually*   **jñ** usually pronounced as *gya*

Guide Courtesy of Yoga International

Additional Resources

Books and Online Sources that contributed to
The Daily Guide To the Yoga Sūtras

Four Chapters on Freedom: Commentary on the Yoga Sūtras of Sage Patanjali by Swami Satyananda Saraswati

Inside the Yoga Sūtras: A Comprehensive Sourcebook for the Study and Practice of Patanjali's Yoga Sūtras by Reverend Jaganath Carrera

Simple-yoga.org: an online resource for yoga classes, philosophy, and in-person retreats.

That is This: Patanjali's Yoga Sūtras Padas 2 and 3 by Anand Mehrotra

The Yoga Sūtras of Patañjali: A New Edition, Translation, and Commentary by Edwin F. Bryant

The Yoga Sūtras of Patanjali: Translation and Commentary by Swami Satchidananda

This Is That: Patanjali's Yoga Sūtras Padas 1 and 2 by Anand Mehrotra

YouTube: *Yogic Gurukul*

YouTube: *Academy of Indian Philosophy*

Recommended Books and Publications for Study

Autobiography of a Yogi by Paramahansa Yogananda

Breath by James Nestor

Body by Breath by Jill Miller

Haṭha Yoga Pradīpikā by Swami Muktibodhananda

I Am That by Nisargadatta Maharaj

Light on Life by B.K.S. Iyengar – a classic text on yoga philosophy and practice

Light on Yoga B.K.S. Iyengar

Living with the Himalayan Masters by Swami Rama

Mindfulness in Plain English by Bhante Gunaratana

Peace is Every Step by Thich Nhat Hanh

Spiritual Graffiti, by MC Yogi

Think Like a Monk by Jay Shetty

The Art of Happiness by Dalai Lama

The Bhagavad Gita for Daily Living: A Verse-by-Verse Commentary by Eknath Easwaran

The Breathing Book by Donna Farhi

The Divine Romance by Paramahansa Yogananda

The Power of Now by Eckhart Tolle

The Science of Breath by Swami Rama

The Yoga of Breath by Richard Rosen

Yoga Journal Magazine

Yoga Nidra Scripts by Tamara Skyhawk (Verma)

Online Yoga Resources and Apps

365 Days of Meditation: Meditations to help you feel more relaxed, inspired, connected, and empowered to choose to live a healthier, more joyful, and meaningful life.

AuthenticStrengths.com: At Authentic Strengths Advantage® you can leverage the science of positive psychology to discover your strengths and download your unique strengths profile for FREE. Empower your personal and professional life for sustainable, positive change!

BohoBeautiful.life: Inspiring yoga, fitness, and travel journeys to nourish the mind, body, and soul.

Calm.com: Join former monk, purpose coach, and best-selling author Jay Shetty on a journey to take positive action toward the life of your dreams.

Chopra.com: A holistic hub for wellness wisdom, meditation guidance, and in-person retreats to elevate your life.

Danielroqueo.com Daniel Roquéo is a Spiritual Teacher and the founder of The Path To Freedom App and the Freedom Tribe Family—a Loving, Thriving and Supportive spiritual family and community where individuals get to connect with one another, hang out in High Minded Fellowship for mutual support. His teachings empower individuals to transform their lives, setting themselves free from fear, worry, doubt, a sense of lack, scarcity, separation, and the feeling of not being enough.

davidji.com: davidji is a globally recognized mindbody health & wellness expert, mindful performance trainer, meditation teacher and author of three award-winning books: Sacred Powers: The Five Secrets to Awakening Transformation; Destressifying: The Real-World Guide to Personal Empowerment, Lasting Fulfillment, and Peace of Mind; and Secrets of Meditation: A Practical Guide to Inner Peace & Personal Transformation. davidji has taught millions of people around the world to heal their hearts, plant powerful intentions and manifest their dream lives. His grasp of time tested solutions combined with real-world practical applications, have helped people at every life stage and circumstance find balance, heal deep wounds, and transform into their best versions.

GaiaMeditation.com: An online resource for meditation.

Glo.com: An online platform for yoga classes and wellness resources.

Great Meditation: An online resource for meditation.

Headspace.com: A meditation app with guided meditations and mindfulness resources.

InnerDimensiontv.com: Yoga, meditation and daily wisdom focused on the 6 human dimensions to awaken your full potential.

InsightTimer.com: A popular meditation app with thousands of free guided meditations and mindful resources.

Kyrian.Art: Owner Niccolò Angeli, from Tuscany, Italy created Academia infinita an online school for spirituality that includes meditations, courses, and other engaging spiritual content.

Mooji.org: Video and audio recordings of Mooji's Satsangs can be found at *www. mooji.org/mooji-tv* and *www.mooji.org/sahaja-express*.

OmniMindfulness.com: Holistic Mindfulness Coach, Social Media Strategist and Podcast. Blends ancient Indian Vedic wisdom with modern mindfulness techniques. Specializing in supporting high-functioning professional women, Shilpa provides a unique fusion of spiritual wisdom and tech-savvy marketing strategies, guiding women through the complexities of entrepreneurial life while maintaining holistic life harmony.

PalouseMindfulness.com: MBSR Mindfulness-Based Stress Reduction program FREE online 8-week course founded by Jon Kabat-Zinn.

SattvaConnect.com: A traditional yogic program online with over 1,000 classes, lectures, and programs directly from the banks of the Ganges in Rishikesh, India.

Spotify: A music app to find yoga music and create playlists.

Wanderlust.tv: An online yoga platform featuring some of the best yoga teachers in the industry.

WimHofMethod.com: A website for learning the Wim Hof Method of breathing and cold exposure. Find out about the free App to experience the life-changing techniques.

YogaInternational.com: A comprehensive website for yoga articles, classes, and resources.

YogaJournal.com: A popular magazine and online resource for yoga practitioners and teachers.

Yogananda.org: Learn the sacred science of Kriya Yoga meditation to transform and bring balance to your life.

Retreat Centers, Yoga Schools, Festivals

Akhanda Yoga Institue: Akhandā Yoga Institute was founded by Himalayan Master Yogrishi Vishvketu to support people in realizing their unique, individual potential. 'Akhanda' means whole and indivisible, and Akhanda Yoga Institute supports people in their quest to achieve wholeness. Our expertise lies in using time-honoured tools to nurture self-healing, support balanced self-development, and help people realize their unique, individual potential.We share wellbeing with the world by offering authentic, proven techniques and a holistic toolkit of Yogic practices, including: Asana | Prāṇāyāma | Mantra | Meditation | Yogic Philosophy. Website: *akhandayoga.com*

Bhakti Fest: An annual music and yoga festival held in Joshua Tree, California, and other international sites. Website: *bhaktifest.com*

Chopra Center: Features meditation, yoga, nutrition, and mental well-being, aimed at helping individuals achieve a balanced and healthy lifestyle. Additionally, the site provides information about Chopra-certified programs and events designed to enhance overall well-being. Website: *Chopra.com*

Himalayan Institute: Founded by Swami Rama, author of "Living with the Himalayan Masters." A world leader in the field of yoga, meditation, spirituality, and holistic health. The Himalayan Institute is a non-profit international organization dedicated to serving humanity through educational, spiritual, and humanitarian programs. Website: *himalayaninstitute.org*

International Yoga Festival: The annual IYF, organized by Parmarth Niketan in the sacred and heavenly Rishikesh, India, the birthplace of Yoga and Yoga Capital of the World. website: *internationalyogafestival.org*

Mooji.org: Video and audio recordings of Mooji's Satsangs can be found at *www.mooji.org/mooji-tv* and *www.mooji.org/sahaja-express*.

Prana Vinyasa Yoga School: Movement, meditation and life regeneration for all. Website: *ShivaRea.com*

Red House Wellness offers programs and resources for transformational experiences to reclaim your health, happiness and purpose. Download FREE resources to achieve lasting change. Website: *Redhousewellness.com*

Sattva Yoga Academy: Offers yoga training in traditional Himalayan Kundalini Yoga in Rishikesh, India. Website: *sattvayogaacademy.com*

Self-Realization Fellowship: A worldwide religious organization founded in 1920 by Paramahansa Yogananda, author of <u>Autobiography of a Yogi</u>. Website: *yogananda.org*

SRMD Yoga: Rooted in spirituality, SRMD Yoga nourishes the body, centres the mind, and enables you to make the most of every moment. Welcome to the ultimate journey of well-being.Website: *srmdyoga.org*

Triguna Yoga: An exceptional, eclectic and all-encompassing yoga program offering 200 hr and 300 hr RYS training in Rishikesh, India. No matter if you are a beginner, experienced or whether you want to start a career in teaching Yoga or not this is the perfect training right from the river Ganges.
Website: *TrigunaYoga.net*

Vipassana: A popular 10-day silent meditation retreat with centers worldwide. Website: *www.dhamma.org*

Wake Up and Manifest Yoga Training: Online yoga training with the author of *The Daily Guide to the Yoga Sūtras*. By application only and limited to 8 participants. Website: *Yogaawakeningwithsue.com*

Music

Kirtan and Kundalini: A sacred music and yoga school founded by Snatam & Sopurkh offering live mantra and kundalini yoga & meditation classes. They also offer online courses and 40-day meditations. You can also learn kirtan and take harmonium and tabla lessons. Website: *www.kirtanandkundalini.com*

Krishna Das: An online resource for Bhakti Yoga and Kirtan. Website: *krishnadas.com*

Mike Cohen Kirtan: An online resource for learning to play harmonium. Website: *mikecohenkirtan.com*

Mooji Mala Music: A collection of music from Heart Satsangs with Mooji. YouTube channel: *youtube.com/c/MoojiMalaMusic*

Sunreed Instruments: Source for Sound Healing® Changing Lives Through Sound™ Crystal Singing Bowls, Traditional Native American Drums, Rattles, and so much more*!* Website: *sunreed.com*

Endnotes

1 - Touskova, T. P. (2022). A novel Wim Hof psychophysiological training program to reduce stress responses during an Antarctic expedition. *Journal of International Medical Research*. https://doi.org/https://journals.sagepub.com/doi/full/10.1177/03000605221089883

2 - Worth, N. (2014). *The Enlightenment of the Body: The Theory and Practice of Winds and Channels Yoga at Namdroling Monastery and Nunnery in South India* [Doctor of Philosophy]. https://libraetd.lib.virginia.edu/downloads/sf268601m?filename=1_Worth_Naomi_2022_PHD.pdf

3 - Subbarayappa, B. (1971). *Science in India: A Concise History of Science in India* (p. 168). Sage Journals. https://journals.sagepub.com/doi/abs/10.1177/002182867500600207?journalCode=jhaa

4 - Udupa, K., & Sathyaprabha, T. (2014). Influence of Yoga on the Autonomic Nervous System. *IGI Global*. https://doi.org/https://www.igi-global.com/chapter/influence-of-yoga-on-the-autonomic-nervous-system/187467

5 - Quote – Anand Ji That Is This: Patanjali's Yoga Sūtras Padas 3 and 4 (Kindle Locations 2319-2321). Sattva Publication. Kindle Edition.

Mehrotra, A. (2020). *This Is That – Patanjali's Yoga Sūtras Padas 1 and 2*. Sattva Publications PVT. LTD. https://doi.org/https://www.amazon.com/THIS-THAT-Patanjalis-Sūtras-Padas/dp/8193988213

Illustration Credits

Cover Image: mandalaking/Shutterstock.com
Cover Yoga Body: Vector_100/Shutterstock.com
Half, full, and number mandalas throughout book: mandalaking/Shutterstock.com
Title Page Yoga Body: Vector_100/Shutterstock.com
1.2 to 1.4: Pogaryts'kyy/Shutterstock.com
1.5 to 1.11: Transia Design/Shutterstock.com
1.12 to 1.15: Pogaryts'kyy/Shutterstock.com
1.16 to 1.23: Gorbash Varvara/Shutterstock.com
1.23: Pogaryts'kyy/Shutterstock.com
1.24 to 1.29: Katika/Shutterstock.com
1.29: Viktoriia_M/Shutterstock.com
1.30 to 1.32: anvinoart/Shutterstock.com
1.33 to 1.40: Gorbash Varvara/Shutterstock.com
1.41 to 1.51: Gorbash Varvara/Shutterstock.com
2.1 to 2.2: Pogaryts'kyy/Shutterstock.com
2.3 to 2.9: Pogaryts'kyy/Shutterstock.com
2.10 to 2.17: yulianas/Shutterstock.com
2.18 to 2.19: Veronika By/Shutterstock.com
2.20 to 2.25: Katika/Shutterstock.com
2.20 to 2.25: Shafran/Shutterstock.com
2.26 to 2.27: RaSveta/Shutterstock.com
2.28 to 2.56: Amovitania/Shutterstock.com
2.33 to 2.39: IB Photography/Shutterstock.com
2.40 to 2.45: Rusyn/Shutterstock.com
2.46 to 2.48: Pogaryts'kyy/Shutterstock.com
2.49 to 2.53: SinceALuck16/Shutterstock.com
2.54 to 2.55: Pogaryts'kyy/Shutterstock.com

2.55: Manjunatha S/Dreamstime.com

3.1 to 3.3: Peratek/Shutterstock.com

3.1: Vanilladesign/Dreamstime.com

3.2: Zsschreiner/Shutterstock.com

3.3: Pogaryts'kyy/Shutterstock.com

3.4 to 3.8: Robindranath Debnath/Shutterstock.com

3.9 to 3.15: Hellocho/Shutterstock.com

3.12: Prabir Bhattacharjee/Dreamstime.com

3.16 to 3.49: Williams Melo/Shutterstock.com

3.16 to 3.26: Gorbash Varvara/Shutterstock.com

3.24: anvinoart/Shutterstock.com

3.25: anvinoart/Shutterstock.com

3.27 to 3.29: Atatay/Shutterstock.com

3.30 to 3.39: yulianas/Shutterstock.com

3.32: REYYARTS/Shutterstock.com

3.40 to 3.45: Gorbash Varvara/Shutterstock.com

3.41: IVANCHINA ANNA/Shutterstock.com

3.46: Allexxe/Shutterstock.com

3.47 to 3.49: Smiling Fox/Shutterstock.com

3.47: Lek Suwarin/Shutterstock.com

3.47: Greenberg_see/Shutterstock.com

3.50 to 3.52: Ka Lina/Shutterstock.com

3.53 to 3.56: RaSveta/Shutterstock.com

3.55: snapgalleria/Shutterstock.com

4.1 to 4.12: Gorbash Varvara/Shutterstock.com

4.13 to 4.21: Gorbash Varvara/Shutterstock.com

4.22 to 4.28: Gorbash Varvara/Shutterstock.com

4.29 to 4.32: Peratek/Shutterstock.com

4.33 to 4.34: Gorbash Varvara/Shutterstock.com

About the Author

Susan Fendler's passion for yoga and music has been the driving force behind her life's work. She grew up in New Hampshire, where she developed a love for the arts at an early age. After graduating from Eastman School of Music, Susan pursued a career in music education and performance in New York.

Despite a fulfilling career as a music educator, Susan felt a calling to explore the world of yoga. She began practicing yoga over 25 years ago and quickly fell in love with the physical and spiritual benefits of the practice.

Susan's love of yoga inspired her to delve deep into yogic philosophy and to study Patanjali's *Yoga Sūtras* in depth. Her commentary on the *Yoga Sūtras* is her gift to her students and practitioners around the world in hopes to simplify and clarify this ancient wisdom. As a master yoga instructor, she has trained numerous students to become certified yoga instructors themselves, passing on her knowledge and passion to others.

When she's not teaching yoga or writing, Susan loves to travel and explore new cultures. She trained in Rishikesh, India at Triguna Yoga Ashram and also in Anusara Yoga in Park City, Utah. One of her favorite places is Bali, Indonesia where she leads yoga retreats. She also enjoys skiing and spends her winters on the slopes in Park City.

Stay Connected

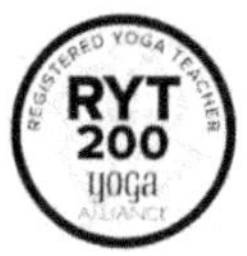

yogaaawakeningwithsue.com/online-yoga-training

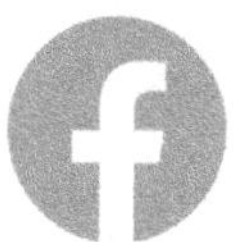

www.facebook.com/Yogaaawakeningwithsue

www.instagram.com/yogaaawakeningwithsue

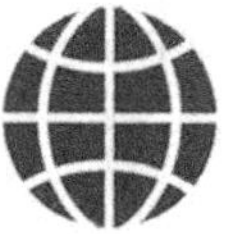

YogaAwakeningwithSue.com

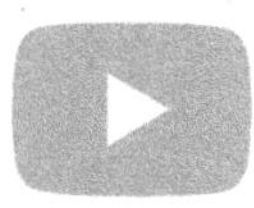

www.youtube.com/@YogaAwakening

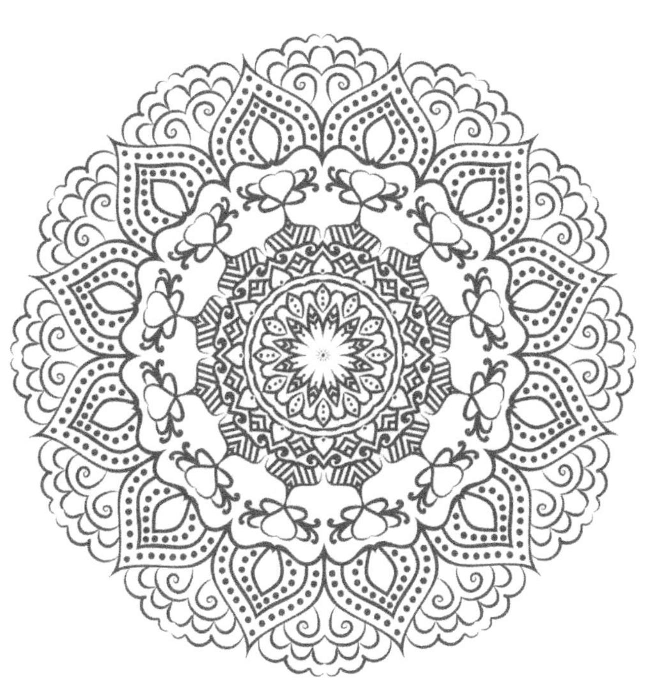